P9-DTP-313

Setting Your Weight

A Complete Program

Fitness, Health & Nutrition was created by Rebus, Inc. and published by Time-Life Books.

REBUS, INC.

Publisher: RODNEY FRIEDMAN
Editorial Director: CHARLES L. MEE JR.

Editor: THOMAS DICKEY
Executive Editor: SUSAN BRONSON
Senior Editor: CARL LOWE
Associate Editors: MARY CROWLEY, WILLIAM DUNNETT
Contributing Editor: JACQUELINE DAMIAN
Copy Editor: LINDA EPSTEIN

Art Director: JUDITH HENRY
Designer: FRANCINE KASS
Photographer: STEVEN MAYS
Photo Stylist: NOLA LOPEZ
Photo Assistant: TIMOTHY JEFFS

Test Kitchen Director: GRACE YOUNG
Recipe Editor: BONNIE J. SLOTNICK
Contributing Editor: MARYA DALRYMPLE
Chief of Research: CARNEY W. MIMMS III
Assistant Editor: PENELOPE CLARK

Time-Life Books Inc. is a wholly owned subsidiary of

TIME INCORPORATED

Founder: HENRY R. LUCE 1898-1967

Editor-in-Chief: JASON MCMANUS
Chairman and Chief Executive Officer: J. RICHARD MUNRO
President and Chief Operating Officer: N.J. NICHOLAS JR.
Corporate Editor: RAY CAVE
Executive Vice President, Books: KELSO F. SUTTON
Vice President, Books: GEORGE ARTANDI

TIME-LIFE BOOKS INC.

Editor: GEORGE CONSTABLE

Executive Editor: ELLEN PHILLIPS
Director of Design: LOUIS KLEIN
Director of Editorial Resources: PHYLLIS K. WISE
Editorial Board: RUSSELL B. ADAMS JR., DALE M.
BROWN, ROBERTA CONLAN, THOMAS H. FLAHERTY, LEE
HASSIG, DONIA ANN STEELE, ROSALIND STUBENBERG,
KIT VAN TULLEKEN, HENRY WOODHEAD
Director of Photography and Research: JOHN CONRAD
WEISER

President: CHRISTOPHER T. LINEN
Chief Operating Officer: JOHN M. FAHEY JR.
Senior Vice President: JAMES L. MERCER
Vice Presidents: STEPHEN L. BAIR, RALPH J. CUOMO,
NEAL GOFF, STEPHEN L. GOLDSTEIN, JUANITA T.
JAMES, HALLETT JOHNSON III, CAROL KAPLAN, SUSAN J.
MARUYAMA, ROBERT H. SMITH, PAUL R. STEWART,
JOSEPH J. WARD
Director of Production Services: ROBERT J. PASSANTINO

Editorial Operations
Copy Chief: DIANE ULLIUS
Production: CELIA BEATTIE
Library: LOUISE D. FORSTALL

FITNESS, HEALTH & NUTRITION

Setting Your Weight
A Complete Program

Time-Life Books, Alexandria, Virginia

CONSULTANTS FOR THIS BOOK

Theodore B. Van Itallie, M.D., Professor of Medicine at the College of Physicians and Surgeons, Columbia University, is codirector of the Obesity Research Center at St. Luke's-Roosevelt Hospital Center/Rockefeller University, New York City.

Ann Grandjean, Ed.D., is Associate Director of the Swanson Center for Nutrition, Omaha, Neb.; chief nutrition consultant to the U.S. Olympic Committee; and an instructor in the Sports Medicine Program, Orthopedic Surgery Department, University of Nebraska Medical Center.

Myron Winick, M.D., is the R.R. Williams Professor of Nutrition, Professor of Pediatrics, Director of the Institute of Human Nutrition, and Director of the Center for Nutrition, Genetics and Human Development at Columbia University College of Physicians and Surgeons. He has served on the Food and Nutrition Board of the National Academy of Sciences and is the author of many books, including *Your Personalized Health Profile*.

Colonel Frederick R. Drews, who designed the exercise routines on pages 48-49 and 80-81, is a Doctor of Physical Education who directs the Army Physical Fitness Research Institute at the U.S. Army War College in Carlisle, Pennsylvania. He is the author of *A Healthy Life: Exercise, Behavior, Nutrition*.

For information about any Time-Life book please call 1-800-621-7026, or write:
Reader Information
Time-Life Customer Service
P.O. Box C-32068
Richmond, Virginia 23261-2068

Library of Congress Cataloging-in-Publication Data
Setting your weight.
(Fitness, health & nutrition)
Includes index.
1. Reducing diets. I. Time-Life Books. II. Series: Fitness, health, and nutrition.
RM222.2.S45 1988   613.2'5   87-31422
ISBN 0-8094-6191-9
ISBN 0-8094-6192-7 (lib. bdg.)

Contents

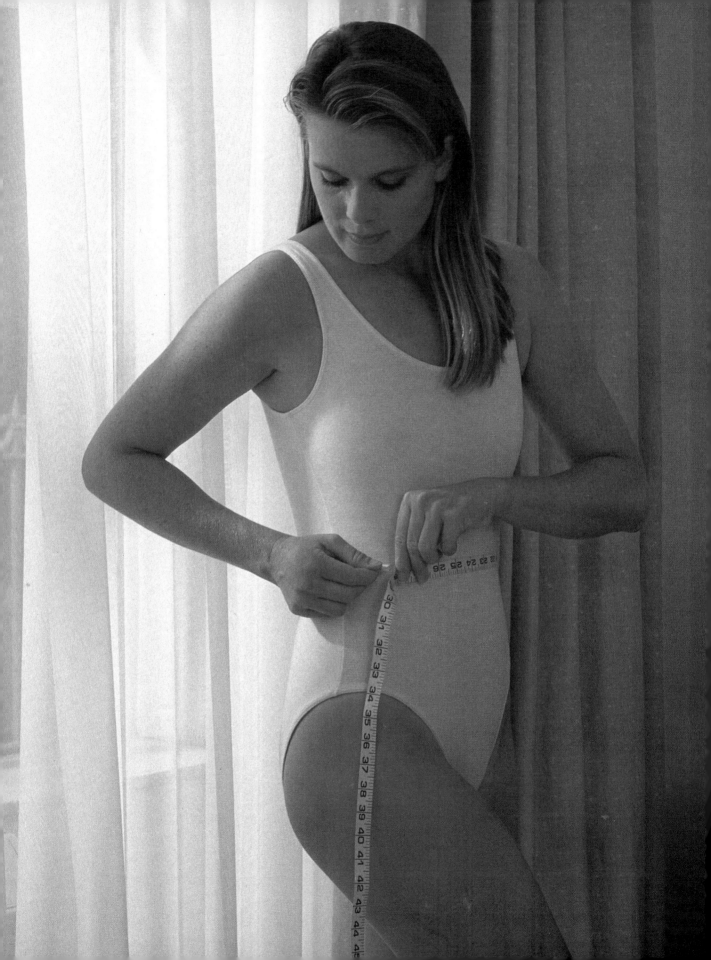

CHAPTER ONE

The Essentials of Weight Control

Why excess pounds accumulate — and the right plan for taking them off

To lose weight safely and permanently, you need to alter both your eating habits and your exercise habits. In the long run, weight-loss programs that stress only what you eat and that place you on special diets that differ radically from what you normally eat do not produce long-term weight loss.

That is why this is not a diet book — at least not in the sense that it provides a regimen for a rapid weight loss that you follow for a limited time only. Researchers studying subjects who have tried special diets — other than those administered in hospital settings — have found that such programs seldom result in a permanent reduction in pounds. As a rule, these diets may allow you to slim down, but after you resume your previous eating habits, your lost weight will return, often accompanied by extra pounds you did not have before. To avoid this difficulty, you must change your daily routines, particularly what you eat and how active you are, and adopt practices you can adhere to for the rest of your life.

Energy Balance: The Key to Gain and Loss

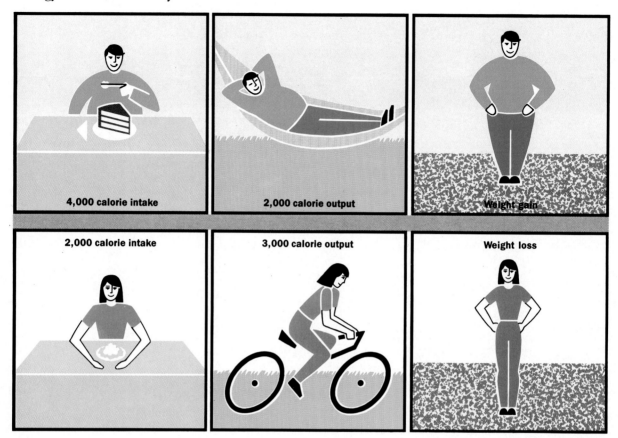

4,000 calorie intake

2,000 calorie output

Weight gain

2,000 calorie intake

3,000 calorie output

Weight loss

When your energy intake (supplied by food) is in balance with your energy output (expended to sustain daily activities), your weight stays relatively stable. However, when intake is greater than output — as measured in calories — the excess calories are stored as body fat and you will gain weight *(top)*. To lose weight, you need to tip this energy balance by consuming fewer calories and increasing your physical activity until output exceeds intake. Your body will then turn to the stored fat for energy, causing weight loss *(bottom)*.

What causes you to become overweight?

The energy contained in the food you consume — which your body absorbs and uses to maintain its internal functions and power its day-to-day activities, including exercise — is the most important variable affecting your weight. When you eat foods that contain more energy than necessary to fuel your body and repair its structure, the metabolic processing of the excess nutrients results in the creation of body fat. The nutrients enter your bloodstream through the walls of your stomach or intestines, and instead of taking part in the chemical reactions that produce energy, these substances — whether they were originally dietary protein, carbohydrate or fat — are used to synthesize triglycerides, which are stored as body fat.

So the formula that produces significant weight loss and long-term maintenance of a desirable lower weight is a decrease in the amount of food energy you eat accompanied by an increase in the energy your activities use up. Those changes in energy balance deprive your body of excess food energy it might store as fat and force it to draw on some of the energy stored in the fat that has already been accumulated.

Why should you control your weight?

Body fat, contained in adipose tissue, puts increased stress on your ligaments, tendons, bones and lean muscle tissue, which has to support the fat's weight. Keeping your weight down avoids this burden and makes it easier for you to move around during normal activities as well as during workouts. And being reasonably slender can benefit your back. Excess fat is often carried at the front of the abdomen, which can create a forward tug on the backbone. Losing that fat and keeping it off reduces this stressful pull.

While the exact physiological mechanisms that endow slim people with better health are not well understood, statistical studies of population groups have established that weighing less better enables you to undergo surgery without medical complications and, if you are a woman, to give birth more safely. Data compiled by life insurance companies show that American men who are obese (20 percent heavier than the statistical average) have a 20 percent shorter life expectancy than the norm. Obese women have a 10 percent shorter life expectancy than average women.

Many long-term studies have also shown that high-fat diets and excess weight are significant risk factors for a whole spectrum of life-threatening diseases, including hypertension, stroke, diabetes, gall bladder problems and certain types of cancer. The intake of dietary fat, especially saturated fat, is associated with an elevated blood cholesterol level, a major factor in coronary heart disease.

For the overweight person, thick layers of insulating fat increase discomfort in hot weather. Normally, a significant amount of heat escapes from the body as the blood circulates through tissues just under the skin. But extra layers of fat tissue under the skin block this dissipation of heat. And, because overweight people radiate less heat than thin people do, they perspire more heavily to give off body heat through the evaporation of moisture from their skin.

In addition, according to today's standards of physical beauty, it is better to be slim than heavy, and there is a strong social stigma attached to being fat. Many people regard those who are overweight as weak-willed. Studies by social scientists have found that heavier people may have more trouble getting a job than their thinner counterparts, their social interactions may be less satisfactory and their self-image and self-respect may suffer. In some instances, losing weight can alleviate those problems and make an important difference in how you see yourself and how others see you.

How do calories affect your weight?

The amount of energy contained in your food and the amount of energy used by your body are commonly expressed in calories. One calorie equals the amount of energy necessary to raise a kilogram of water one degree Celsius. Only carbohydrates, fats and proteins contain calories. Water, fiber, vitamins and minerals do not contain any. (Because of variations in storage facilities, handling methods and the conditions in which a food item was grown or raised, calorie counts for the same item may differ from one reading to the next.)

The amount of energy necessary to form a pound of adipose tissue is approximately 3,500 calories. Therefore, to lose a pound of fat-containing tissue, you have to burn up 3,500 more calories than you consume in your food.

Can't you just consume fewer calories in order to lose weight?
Trying to lose pounds by eating less can cause weight loss. However, that strategy is not as effective for long-term weight reduction and maintenance of a lower weight as is a program that combines exercise with a calorie-restricted diet.

Studies show that when you reduce dietary calories, your body may lower its resting metabolic rate, managing to get by on fewer calories. The result is that after a short period of dieting you will have to restrict your food intake even more to lose weight than you did at the beginning of your diet. And if you are eating a severely limited amount of food, you are more likely to stop dieting. However, research on athletes and the overweight demonstrates that exercising burns up more calories and allows you to eat more food while still maintaining a caloric deficit between the amount you eat and the amount you use in daily activity.

Another problem you may confront if you try to lose weight solely by means of calorie restriction is that your body will not merely use its own fat for energy; it will also burn a significant amount of muscle tissue to supply its energy needs. This is undesirable since it is your excess fat, not your lean tissue, that is related to problems like hypertension and diabetes (although researchers have not isolated the mechanisms by which it contributes to these life-threatening conditions). Studies of dieters show that those who work out lose less muscle tissue and a higher percentage of fat than those who are inactive.

What kind of exercise is the best for losing weight?
Any regular exercise routine that you find convenient is probably suitable. However, to burn the most calories per minute, you have to perform an aerobic exercise — like running, cycling or brisk walking — that involves the repeated motion of the large muscle groups in the arms or legs. These endurance activities can be sustained for relatively long periods and so can burn up more calories than anaerboic exercises, such as weight lifting or sprinting, which are performed more intensely but for much shorter periods. Moreover, researchers have found that an aerobic exercise performed for at least 20 minutes draws on fat for at least 50 percent of its energy. Anaerobic activities, on the other hand, draw more heavily on glycogen, the starch stored in the muscles and liver, to fuel their motion.

Won't exercising make you hungrier and liable to eat more?
Contrary to what you might expect, studies show that an intense

exercise session tends to decrease your appetite and cause you to eat less at your next meal than you normally would. And, while it is true that if you follow a consistent exercise program you may increase your total food intake, your energy output may more than compensate. A study of middle-aged joggers found that even though they consistently consumed more calories daily than their sedentary counterparts, they weighed less than the men and women in the study who did not exercise.

Does shedding excess pounds reverse the health hazards of being overweight?

Losing weight does mitigate the health risks associated with being overweight; moreover, studies have established that you do not have to lose a large amount of weight to improve your health. For instance, a loss of as little as five pounds can significantly lower the blood-sugar level of some diabetics. And similarly small weight losses have been shown to lower elevated blood cholesterol levels and blood pressure, important indicators of cardiovascular health.

Is all fat unhealthy?

No. In fact, you cannot live without some fat. Carbohydrates and fat are your main sources of energy for the metabolic processes that keep you alive and enable you to move around. But by weight, fat is the most energy-dense source of fuel; it supplies twice as much energy per pound as carbohydrates. This is possible because most of your fat consists of triglycerides, chemicals whose molecular construction makes them efficient energy-storage centers. Digestive and metabolic processes convert dietary fat to body fat.

When you perform a low-intensity exercise like slow jogging, your body gets about half of its energy from its carbohydrate reserves and about half from its reserves of fat (as well as a small amount from protein). But when you run or exercise for two hours or more, you exhaust most of your carbohydrate reserves. Your body must then rely mainly on its fat reserves to provide muscular energy.

In addition to its role as fuel for movement and exercise, essential fat, which is located in your muscle tissue, heart, lungs, liver and other organs, takes part in these organs' necessary physiological functions by absorbing, storing and transporting the fat-soluble vitamins (A, D, E and K). These vitamins, dissolved in essential fat, are catalysts for vital metabolic functions such as the creation of blood-clotting factors in the liver. Ingested fat also supplies essential fatty acids and helps delay stomach emptying so that digestion can take place. Finally, essential fat forms the outer protective covering of nerves and is needed in cell membranes.

Women normally have a larger proportion of essential fat than men because they have fat deposited in the breasts, upper thighs, hips and buttocks. This extra fat is necessary for reproduction and provides energy used in the production of milk for nursing.

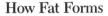

How Fat Forms

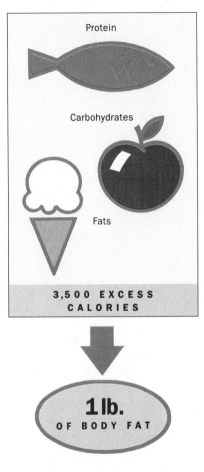

Body fat forms not only from dietary fat, but from protein and carbohydrates as well. Though dietary fat contains more calories per gram than the other two nutrients, any food supplying calories not burned up in daily activity will be converted into fat. An excess of 3,500 calories — whether consumed over a week or a year — will increase body fat by approximately one pound.

What Happens to Fat Cells

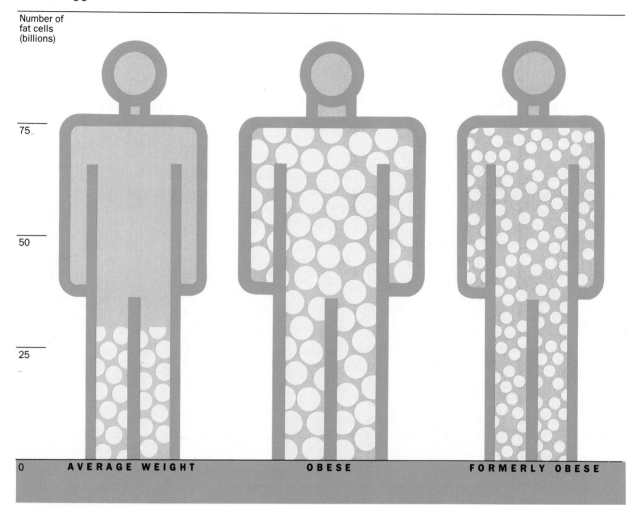

Number of
fat cells
(billions)

75

50

25

0

AVERAGE WEIGHT   **OBESE**   **FORMERLY OBESE**

A person of average weight has one third as many fat cells as an obese person *(left and center)* — 25 to 30 billion fat cells as compared to 75 billion. The average amount of fat within each fat cell is about 35 percent greater in the obese. Any weight loss occurs solely through a decrease in cell size *(far right)*, and when the obese lose weight, their fat cells can shrink to about one third the size of cells in nonobese people. The number of fat cells remains the same, however; the cells will expand again if the lost pounds are regained.

What happens to your body when you lose weight?

Researchers studying fat cells believe that while most of those cells are created early in life, overeating as an adult may produce additional fat cells. When you lose weight, the fat cells will shrink as the body draws on their triglyceride content to meet its energy needs. But these cells will not vanish; indeed, they will fill up with triglycerides again if you consume too many calories, causing you to regain the weight you lost.

Some researchers have theorized that this physiological process occurs because of a human evolutionary adaptation. In epochs when famines occurred frequently, human survival may have depended on the body's use of the fat that had been stored when a surplus of food was available. Now that surplus food is generally available all the time in the developed countries of the world, the body's mechanism for storing this fat in adipose tissue has become an impediment to weight loss and a threat to health.

If your parents are fat, will you have to struggle to maintain your optimal weight?

Medical researchers believe that some people have an inherited tendency to be overweight, although scientists do not yet understand the genetic mechanisms by which this occurs. Studies of children raised by adoptive parents show that their weight correlates more strongly with the weight of their biological parents than with the weight of the people who raised them. Also, studies of identical twins, who have inherited identical sets of genes, show that their weights are more closely matched than the weights of fraternal twins, who do not have the same genetic makeup. Nevertheless, while you cannot alter your genes, virtually all weight-control researchers agree that your lifestyle and your eating habits are significant, controllable factors that affect your weight.

Your eating habits — how much you eat, when you eat and what kinds of foods you eat — form a group of behaviors that you originally learned from your parents and your peers. Habits such as always eating everything on your plate or ending your meal with a rich dessert are acquired eating behaviors that can contribute to being overweight. Replacing these habits with others is called behavior modification. Many researchers believe that behavior modification holds the key to weight control for most overweight people, particularly those who have dieted repeatedly but failed to achieve permanent weight loss. With their own efforts and sometimes with professional help, many people can learn new attitudes and eating behaviors.

How do you gauge your energy usage?

Scientists call the minimum rate at which your body uses energy the basal metabolic rate. You reach this basal rate first thing in the morning, before you get started with your daily activities. This rate is the minimum rate of energy use that the body needs to carry out critical functions while at rest. These functions include breathing, maintaining body temperature, circulation, cellular metabolism and glandular activity. The basal metabolic rate for adults varies from 0.8 to 1.4 calories per minute, according to weight, sex, body composition (amount of muscle tissue) and other factors. Your resting metabolic rate, your rate of energy usage when you are relaxing during the day, is only slightly higher than your basal rate.

The highest rate of energy output is called the thermic effect of exercise, or thermogenesis, the scientific term for your increased energy usage when you are actively using your muscles. A 150-pound man whose metabolism uses one calorie per minute during sleep may expend 12 calories a minute during intense exercise like running or swimming. Some researchers also believe that your metabolism remains elevated for several hours after you finish exercising, but this has not been definitely established.

There is another thermic effect, called the thermic effect of food. This term refers to the increased rate of energy usage that takes place for several hours after a meal as your body expends energy to digest your food and move it through the alimentary canal.

If you seem to gain weight easily, is it because your metabolism is sluggish?
If you have a low resting metabolic rate, it is not because your metabolism is inherently sluggish. Instead, it is a matter of having a low level of muscle mass. A low resting metabolic rate can cause you to gain weight more easily and have a harder time losing weight than someone whose metabolic rate is relatively high. A person with more muscle and a high metabolic rate uses up more energy per minute and is less prone to store food energy as fat than someone with a lower rate. This means that the person with a so-called fast metabolism will burn more calories when performing the same activity — even watching TV.

The variability of your body's energy usage reduces the usefulness of a restricted diet as your sole means of losing weight. When you consume fewer calories than normal, your body cuts down its energy use in an effort to conserve the energy it takes from your diet, and your metabolic rate decreases in response. Exactly how it accomplishes this is not clear. But just as the mechanism for storing fat in adipose tissue may have originated as an adaptation to famine, your body's energy-conserving reaction to a restricted diet may also be an evolutionary response designed to ensure survival during periods of food scarcity.

Do you inevitably gain weight as you get older?
Although most people tend to gain weight as they get older, it has not been determined how much of this weight gain is due to decreased physical activity and how much is due to the physiological aspects of aging. Studies have shown that older people generally use up energy at a lower rate than younger people: Basal metabolism drops by approximately four percent during each decade throughout adulthood. This lowered metabolic rate might make more food energy available for creating adipose tissue as you age, even though your calorie intake remains the same.

Are there surgical techniques that can help you lose weight quickly?
For most people, the risks involved in surgery designed to help them lose weight far outweigh the benefits. These drastic measures are suited only to those for whom obesity is life-threatening.

One operation designed to cause weight loss is gastric reduction surgery, a procedure that shrinks the stomach by stapling part of it closed or that fills up part of the stomach with an inflated balloon. After this procedure, it should take less food to make you feel full; overeating will cause nausea. When your appetite and food intake diminish, of course, you will probably lose weight. However, eventu-

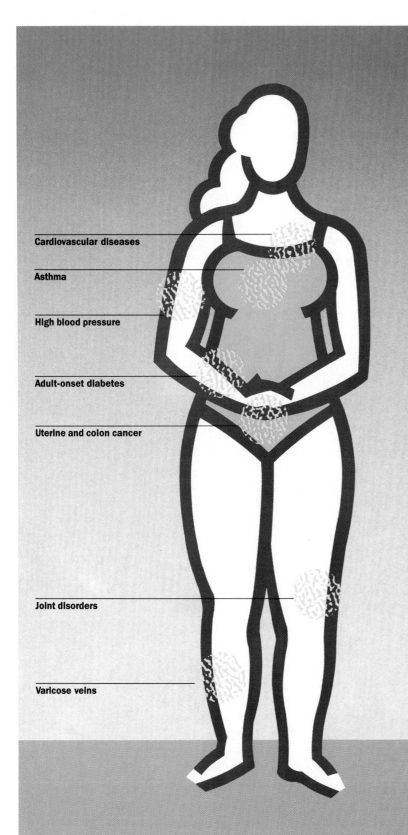

Cardiovascular diseases

Asthma

High blood pressure

Adult-onset diabetes

Uterine and colon cancer

Joint disorders

Varicose veins

Health Risks of Obesity

Doctors have observed for years that obesity is associated with ill health, and clinical evidence for this has been accumulating. The risk of the conditions indicated at left rises when a person exceeds his or her desirable weight by 20 percent.

The most common physical ailment of the obese is hypertension. Those 45 and older are twice as likely to have high blood pressure as their thinner contemporaries; in people younger than 45, the risk is almost six times greater. Many studies have also linked excess body fat with elevated blood cholesterol and increased incidence of heart attack and stroke. Some experts think that the risk of heart disease increases by 30 percent in people who are 20 to 30 percent overweight, and by 100 percent for those who are more than 40 percent overweight. Diabetes is three times more prevalent among the obese, and the American Cancer Society has determined that overweight people are at above average risk for uterine and colon cancer.

The obese are also at greater risk for conditions like asthma, bronchitis, varicose veins, and joint and muscle complaints.

With weight loss, virtually all of these health problems can be reduced or eliminated. For example, in an Australian study, hypertensives who lost an average of 18 pounds saw their blood pressure drop significantly. Among diabetics, losing even a little weight may lower blood sugar levels. And a major study indicated that each 10 percent reduction in weight in men 35-55 years old would result in about a 20 percent decrease in the incidence of coronary heart disease.

Lose Fat, Not Muscle

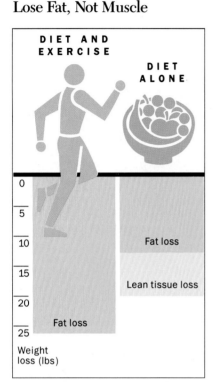

DIET AND EXERCISE

DIET ALONE

Fat loss

Lean tissue loss

Fat loss

0
5
10
15
20
25

Weight loss (lbs)

Combining diet with exercise not only helps promote a more effective loss of body fat, but helps ensure that you lose fat, not muscle mass. In one study, a group that simply reduced food intake lost an average of 20 pounds in two months, while a group that added exercise to their program lost 26 pounds. Furthermore, as the chart above shows, 36 percent of the weight lost in the diet-only group was muscle mass; in the diet-and-exercise group, all the weight lost was fat.

ally your stomach will stretch, allowing you to eat as much as you did before the operation. And some people who have this surgery suffer spleen injury and other complications.

Plastic surgery to suck the fat out from under your skin cannot remove enough fat to benefit the very overweight. In addition, its effects cannot be guaranteed. Studies show that if your eating patterns and lifestyle that caused the build-up of fat continue after the operation, fat that was removed by this procedure, called suction lipectomy, will return.

What is a realistic rate of weight loss?

A realistic goal is to lose between one and two pounds per week. Studies show that people who have taken weight off and kept it off usually lose 1 1/2 pounds per week or less. Gradual weight reduction is more successful than rapid weight loss because it requires only slight changes in behavior that are easier to stick to for a long period of time than are radical changes. In addition, you are more likely to lose fat than muscle when your weight loss is gradual.

Since each pound of adipose tissue represents 3,500 calories, losing a pound a week requires that you burn up one seventh of that amount per day, or at least 500 calories more than you eat. Your calorie deficit should be created by a combination of calorie-burning physical activity and dietary restriction.

Is there a limit to how much weight you can lose?

The set-point theory of weight maintenance contends that for any given level of physical activity, your body has a preset weight and body-fat percentage that it strives to maintain, no matter how much or how little food you eat. Set-point theorists believe that a part of your brain called the hypothalamus orchestrates your metabolism and other internal processes in an effort to stay at this steady set point by varying the rate at which you burn calories.

According to the set-point theory, if your level of physical activity remains constant, merely dieting to lose weight is extremely difficult since your body will slow its metabolic usage of calories to compensate for the reduced supply.

To support the set-point theory, proponents point to the fact that even though Americans consume 10 percent fewer calories than they did 15 years ago, their average weight during that time has increased by about five pounds. What has raised Americans' weight, they claim, is a decrease in activity, not an increase in food, and they hold that obesity is a disease of the sedentary, not of the gluttonous. They believe that exercise is the *only* viable way to control your weight.

However, the advocates of this theory have not been able to identify a specific physiological mechanism by which the hypothalamus or any other part of the body can keep your weight at a particular level. And their theory does not account for the fact that although it is difficult to lose weight by diet alone, it is still possible.

What causes weight-loss plateaus?

Why some dieters reach so-called plateaus, when their weight loss comes to a temporary halt, has not been fully explained, although many weight plateaus may be due to water retention. These plateaus are so common that many researchers in the field consider them to be a normal part of most weight-loss programs. One way to get past a plateau is to increase your weekly exercise and cut back even further on your dietary calories until you begin to lose weight again.

Is it harder for women to lose weight than it is for men?

The fact that many societies expect women to be thinner than men, and that women therefore diet more often to lose weight, may have created the misconception that it is harder for women to lose weight than it is for men. But there is no scientific data to support that notion. Assuming a man and a woman each want to lose the same amount of body fat, neither one has an inborn advantage over the other in their effort to do so.

The same equality, however, does not hold true for weight maintenance. Because women's bodies normally contain a higher percentage of fat and a lower percentage of lean body mass than men's do, in order to maintain a constant, comparable weight, a woman needs to consume fewer calories than a man does. Since the male body consists of a larger proportion of muscle and therefore has a higher metabolic rate than a comparable female body, men may be able to eat more than women without adding adipose tissue.

What is the best way to get rid of cellulite?

Cellulite is a term that was popularized in European spas in the early 20th century to describe unsightly bumps and ripples of fat on the thighs and buttocks. The term was revived in the 1970s, and recent proponents of a cellulite theory argue that this is a special kind of fat, containing water, connective tissue and some kinds of waste products that regular fat lacks. Supposedly, women have more of a problem than men do with cellulite because of their hormonal balance.

However, microscopic comparisons of normal fat tissue with lumpy "cellulite" fat tissue have not established any real difference between the two: Their chemical composition is identical. Lumpy-looking fat occurs when cells containing fat increase in size and bulge out of the connective fiber compartments that usually contain them, giving skin a cross-hatched waffled appearance. But except for differences in appearance, all fat stored in the body's adipose tissue is identical.

Can you control where the fat comes off when you lose weight?

The way in which fat is distributed on your body and the places it comes off when you lose weight are both genetically determined. You cannot spot-reduce by exercising a particular body part or a particular set of muscles.

When you lose weight, the fat deposits that are depleted as your

How Fat Comes Off

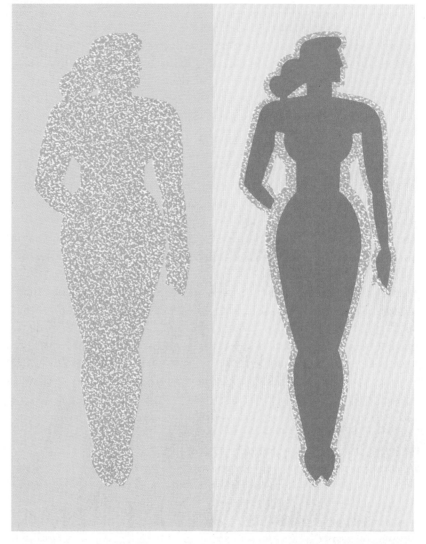

How does body shape change during a weight-loss program? Researchers studied 42 overweight women on a diet-and-exercise regimen. They found that, at each five-pound weight-loss interval, the amount of fat tissue lost in the trunk region was twice that lost in the arms and legs, as shown at right. The study also revealed that fat was lost more quickly in the lower body, particularly the abdomen, hips and buttocks, than in the upper body. Even the wrists and ankles showed reduced measurements after a weight loss of 20 pounds.

body fat decreases are not affected by the type of exercise you perform. Doing exercises like sit-ups for your stomach will strengthen your stomach muscles, but they will not, by themselves, cause fat to disappear from your abdominal area. Eventually, as you follow an exercise and diet program, this and all your adipose tissue will shrink, but spot-reducing exercises, unless they contribute to an overall calorie deficit, will not speed this loss.

How does your body shape change as you lose weight?

Your body measurements do not necessarily change proportionally to the amount of pounds you lose. Research on women who were dieting showed generally that the more pounds these women lost, the more their measurements decreased. On average, the second five pounds they lost reduced their measurements by twice as much as the first five pounds did. This means that their waistline and hip measurements decreased twice as much after the second five pounds they lost as they had after the first five pounds.

Body change during weight loss, therefore, is not a steady, constant process. If you are losing weight and do not immediately see a dramatic difference in your appearance, you should not let that fact demoralize you. Additional weight loss will probably make up for this apparent initial lack of progress.

Will eating particular foods and avoiding others help you lose weight faster?

Basically, the amount of weight you lose or gain comes down to a balance between the amount of calories you eat and the amount you expend. If you eat too much of any kind of food, no matter what its composition or nutritional content, its calories can contribute to your weight gain.

However, protein and carbohydrates are not quite as easily converted into storage fat as are fatty foods — another reason your diet should be low in fat. Furthermore, such complex carbohydrates as the starches in rice, whole-grain products, beans, peas and some vegetables are particularly recommended to dieters because they usually contain a substantial amount of fiber, the indigestible part of plants that has no usable calories because it passes through the body without being absorbed.

Can you lose weight quickly on a high-protein diet?

Diets that allow you to eat large quantities of high-protein, high-fat foods such as meat, eggs and whole milk while restricting your carbohydrate intake periodically gain wide popularity. One reason for their appeal is the rapid weight loss they can produce in a matter of days. Unfortunately, this rapid loss is due mostly to water excretion, not the reduction of body fat. This water loss is caused by two basic metabolic adjustments your body makes when your diet omits carbohydrates. Initially, in order to keep up your blood sugar levels, your body consumes much of your glycogen, the carbohydrates that are stored in your liver and muscles. These carbohydrates are stored in combination with water, and their use results in a large water loss. After about 10 days of adhering to this kind of diet, your body increasingly draws on its fat for energy. However, because carbohydrates are necessary for the complete burning of fat, there is a build-up in the blood of ketone bodies, waste products from incomplete fat oxidation. The excretion of these waste products also uses up water, adding to your apparent weight loss.

A few days after you go off a high-protein diet, you will most likely regain the water you have lost as your body adjusts to the reintroduction of carbohydrates to your diet. Many doctors consider high-protein diets to be dangerous and believe that, through physiological mechanisms not completely understood, the metabolic changes these diets produce can cause serious health problems. In addition, the high fat content of many of these diets has been linked to an increased risk of certain kinds of cancer and cardiovascular problems.

Can you undertake a diet and exercise program at any time?
Almost anyone can go on a diet and begin exercising. If you are extremely overweight, have high blood pressure or are diabetic, you should consult your doctor before trying to lose weight. Anyone who suffers from heart disease or any other condition that requires medical treatment should also seek a doctor's advice before embarking on a weight-loss regimen. Nursing mothers and pregnant women should avoid a restricted-calorie diet, except on the advice of their doctors.

How will this book help you control your weight?
It will give you a program that is practical. The recipes in the following chapters are easy-to-make lowfat, high-carbohydrate dishes that provide an excellent foundation for a diet that allows gradual, permanent weight loss. The ingredients and cooking techniques in these recipes are designed to show you easy ways to cut down on dietary fat, yet prepare dishes that are appetizing and nutritious and that supply generous portions. In addition, this book will guide you toward choosing proper between-meal snacks, dining out sensibly, exercising to burn more calories, and modifying other habits that have probably interfered with your weight control in the past. To start putting these elements together on a day-to-day basis, turn to the next page.

Diets That Don't Work

Roughly half the American adult population is on a weight-loss diet at any one time. But despite the sheer number and seeming variety of popular diets, most of them fall into one of the categories shown at right.

What all these diets promise is quick weight loss with relative ease. That they usually do not deliver is obvious from the high failure rate of dieters: An estimated 75 to 95 percent of people on a diet regain some or all of their lost weight within one or two years of going off their diets. Worse, many of these diets are dangerous because they rely on gimmicks that are deficient in essential vitamins and minerals.

Many diets — especially those that combine high protein or high fat content with low carbohydrates — produce a fluid loss that can fool dieters into thinking they are losing weight rapidly. In fact, the actual fat loss may be quite small, since the body cannot burn fat easily in the absence of carbohydrates. A by-product of this inefficient metabolism is a group of toxic waste products called ketone bodies, which stress, and can eventually damage, the body.

Nutritionists recommend that a reducing diet be nutritionally balanced, with the preponderance of calories coming from carbohydrates. Such a plan is not likely to cause a quick or dramatic weight loss, but the weight that is lost will be mainly excess fat and will stay off permanently if you exercise and do not overeat. The guidelines for a healthy reducing diet, incorporating the recipes in this book, are spelled out on pages 34-39.

TYPE OF DIET	PREMISE	EFFECTS
FASTING	Complete abstinence from eating guarantees weight loss; your body's energy production is not offset by food intake but is supplied instead from the body's own tissues.	Initial weight loss is rapid, but much of the loss is from excretion of water and minerals. Metabolism soon slows to conserve energy, which diminishes rate of weight loss. Fasting also causes significant loss of muscle tissue. This is a drastic weight-loss tactic that should only be attempted by the extremely obese, in a hospital, with medical supervision.
LIQUID PROTEIN	Dieter consumes only a special formula that is very low in calories and so loses weight. The protein content of the formula is supposed to keep the body from losing muscle tissue.	Weight loss may occur, but muscles are not spared as a result of consuming liquid protein. A prepackaged drink is also lacking in other essential nutrients. Possible side effects include nausea, diarrhea and muscle cramps—and the formula may lack important minerals, causing a deficiency that could result in a heart attack.
ONE FOOD	Consumption of one particular food or foods—like grapefruit—causes your body to burn away extra fat.	In addition to being boring and hard to maintain, this diet is nutritionally deficient, since no one food contains all the nutrients necessary for good health. A diet in which fruit is the mainstay, for example, will be low in protein as well as in B vitamins, iron, zinc and calcium.
TIMETABLE	Eating certain foods at specific times or in particular combinations speeds weight loss and improves your health by influencing digestion and absorption of calories and nutrients.	Combining foods in particular ways or eating them only at certain times has no proven effect on calorie utilization or nutrient retention. These diets often emphasize fruit and rice, making them too low in protein for optimal health.
HIGH PROTEIN, HIGH FAT	Restricting carbohydrate consumption while eating large helpings of meat and other fatty foods causes the body to burn fat.	Inclusion of rich foods makes these diets easy to stick to, but a high initial weight drop is due to water loss. In addition, the high-fat content may cause a rise in blood cholesterol, increasing the long-term risk of heart disease. Side effects include fatigue, bad breath and increased stress on liver and kidneys.
HIGH PROTEIN, LOW FAT	Restricting carbohydrate and fat intake while consuming mostly lean foods high in protein causes the body to burn fat.	Initial weight loss is water. This diet has the same side effects as the high-protein, high-fat diet.

How to Design Your Own Program

Successfully setting your weight involves not only losing excess pounds, but maintaining that weight loss. The rest of this chapter will show you the steps to accomplish this.

You will find guidelines on how to estimate your desirable weight; how to control your calorie intake and expenditure to reach that weight; how to plan appetizing low-calorie menus; how to ensure that low-calorie meals are nutritionally balanced; and how to use a food and exercise diary as a tool for achieving your goals. You can then use the following chapters in the book to implement your program.

Begin plotting your program by reviewing the questions at right. The answers will help you analyze why you may be having trouble with your weight and identify some of the habits, attitudes and behaviors you need to focus on to bring your weight under control.

Is your weight under control?

1 Do you think you look overweight?

Standing in front of a mirror can certainly give you a good indication of whether or not you are overweight. But some people have difficulty assessing their weight without the use of an objective guideline. Many of those who are overweight underestimate how much weight they should lose. On the other hand, some people who are actually at their optimal weight think they should be thinner. Experts consider the tables on page 25 the best set of guidelines to showing how much you should weigh for optimal health and longevity.

If you do exceed the recommended weight for your age, height and sex, do not judge yourself too harshly. According to the National Institutes of Health, psychological suffering — including self-blame and feelings of inferiority — is among the most pervasive adverse effects of being overweight. Studies show, however, that losing weight can help produce a positive self-image.

2 Have you lost weight and then regained it?

Many people are successful at losing weight, but keeping it off is another matter. More than three out of four people who lose weight gain it all back in less than a year—in most cases because they tried special diets that they stayed on for only a few weeks. The truth is, a gradual long-term approach to weight-loss makes your program more manageable and is far more realistic in terms of the results you should expect. Although you will probably see some changes in your weight and appearance very quickly using the guidelines in this book, it may take several months before substantial changes are evident.

3 Do you watch television while you eat?

Experts in behavior modification recommend that mealtimes be free of competing activities so that your attention can be on your food. Distractions like watching television can cause you to overeat without even realizing it because they lower your awareness of what you have consumed and how much.

4 Do you eat when you are anxious?

Depending on food to give you an emotional lift can contribute to overeating, especially if the foods you eat to make yourself feel better are high-calorie snack foods like candy or cookies. Your snacks should be low-calorie, high-fiber foods, such as fruits and vegetables, that fill you up with relatively few calories. Or, instead of focusing on eating as a mood lifter, substitute an activity like aerobic exercise, which, studies show, can reduce stress and improve your mood at the same time that it burns calories.

5 | Do you share the misconception of most dieters about which foods are fattening?

Generally, dieters overestimate the fattening effect of the carbohydrates they consume. By weight, sources of carbohydrates like potatoes and pasta are not nearly as high in calories as the butter, creams and sauces that often accompany them. In fact, in a healthy and effective weight-loss program, about 60 percent of the calories in your diet should come from carbohydrates — a guideline used in developing the recipes in this book.

6 | Do you drink alcohol every day?

Alcohol provides no necessary nutrients, but it does contain seven calories per gram, which is more than either carbohydrates or protein provide. For every 12-ounce beer or six-ounce glass of wine you eliminate from your diet daily, you will save approximately 150 calories. Over a year those saved calories would be enough to account for more than 15 lost pounds. For tips on lower-calorie beverages, see the box on page 77.

7 | Can you recall what you ate yesterday?

Without an accurate accounting of when and where you eat, you can easily miscalculate your present food intake, making it difficult to pinpoint the eating habits that are causing you to gain weight. Using a diary like the one on page 41 provides a tangible record. You should keep this diary to analyze your current eating patterns before you start your weight-loss program and then use it to track your progress as you lose weight.

How fast should you lose weight?

You should lose one to two pounds per week. Any loss greater than that will probably be the result of a highly restrictive program that you will not be able to maintain for very long. An extremely rapid weight loss is usually from large water losses rather than loss of fat. As soon as you go off a diet that causes water loss, you quickly regain those pounds of liquid. Furthermore, if you are losing more than two pounds a week through dieting, you are probably not getting the nutrients you need to stay healthy.

For each pound you shed, you need to create a deficit of approximately 3,500 calories between the calories you eat and the calories you use up in activity. Therefore, to lose about a pound per week, you need to use up 500 more calories per day in physical activity than you consume in your food. The calorie charts for foods and activities in this book will guide you toward creating that deficit.

Your Optimal Weight

The most accurate assessment of your ideal weight takes into account your body composition — how much of your weight is lean body mass (muscle and bone) and how much is body fat. For optimum health, body fat should be no more than 20 percent of total body weight for men or 30 percent for women. However, to determine body composition accurately requires both professional analysis and sophisticated equipment. A simpler and more convenient guideline to optimal weight is the Metropolitan Life Insurance height/weight table devised in 1959.

This table, shown on the opposite page, is based on information about body weight and longevity collected from nearly five million Americans over a period of more than 20 years. Optimal weight is the weight at which people in the study lived the longest. The insurance company reassessed these guidelines in 1983 and, using more recent data, released new tables whose optimal weights for men and women of medium height averaged five percent higher than the 1959 weights. But a study by researchers at Harvard University determined that the original weights are preferable. According to the researchers, the 1983 tables underemphasize the benefit of being thin, largely because they do not adjust for the smokers they include. People who smoke tend to be both thinner and die younger than the general population. The presence of the smokers diminished the benefits of being thin, and this accounted for at least a 10 percent increase in optimal weight in some of the lower weight ranges. In fact, when the Harvard researchers examined statistics on people who had never smoked, they found that nonsmokers who weighed 80 to 90 percent of the average weight for Americans had the lowest death rate — a weight well below the 1983 tables, but consistent with the 1959 tables.

To use these tables, you need to know your height and frame size. People with a larger frame can carry slightly more weight without risk. One of the easiest and most accurate ways to determine frame size is to use the measurement of the bone in your elbow. Directions for doing so are on the opposite page along with the chart.

Desirable Weights

HEIGHT	WEIGHT		
	Small Frame	Medium Frame	Large Frame
5'2"	112-120	118-129	126-141
5'3"	115-123	121-133	129-144
5'4"	118-126	124-136	132-148
5'5"	121-129	127-139	135-152
5'6"	124-133	130-143	138-156
5'7"	128-137	134-147	142-161
5'8"	132-141	138-152	147-166
5'9"	136-145	142-156	151-170
5'10"	140-150	146-160	155-174
5'11"	144-154	150-165	159-179
6'0"	148-158	154-170	164-184
6'1"	152-162	158-175	168-189
6'2"	156-167	162-180	173-194
6'3"	160-171	167-185	178-199
6'4"	164-175	172-190	182-204

WOMEN

HEIGHT	WEIGHT		
	Small Frame	Medium Frame	Large Frame
4'10"	92-98	96-107	104-119
4'11"	94-101	98-110	106-122
5'0"	96-104	101-113	109-125
5'1"	99-107	104-116	112-128
5'2"	102-110	107-119	115-131
5'3"	105-113	110-122	118-134
5'4"	108-116	113-126	121-138
5'5"	111-119	116-130	125-142
5'6"	114-123	120-135	129-146
5'7"	118-127	124-139	133-150
5'8"	122-131	128-143	137-154
5'9"	126-135	132-147	141-158
5'10"	130-140	136-151	145-163
5'11"	134-144	140-155	149-168
6'0"	138-148	144-159	153-173

Note: Height for men is in shoes with 1-inch heels; height for women is with 2-inch heels. Weight for both includes indoor clothing.

Measuring Your Frame Size

You can estimate the size of your skeletal frame using your elbow breadth: the distance between the two bones on either side of your elbow. To determine this distance, hold one arm straight out in front of you and raise your hand with your palm turned toward you until your elbow forms a 90-degree angle. In this position, the bones on either side stick out prominently. You can measure the distance between them by placing your elbow on a ruler and visually lining up the outer edge of each bone with a point on the ruler. Then check the column at right, which shows — according to height — the measurements that correspond to a medium frame. Measurements lower than these figures indicate a small frame; higher elbow widths indicate a large frame.

HEIGHT (in 1" heels)	ELBOW BREADTH Medium Frame
Men	
5'2"-5'3"	2½"-2⅞"
5'4"-5'7"	2⅝"-2⅞"
5'8"-5'11"	2¾"-3"
6'0"-6'3"	2¾"-3⅛"
6'4"	2⅞"-3¼"
Women	
4'10"-4'11"	2¼"-2½"
5'0"-5'3"	2¼"-2½"
5'4"-5'7"	2⅜"-2⅝"
5'8"-5'11"	2⅜"-2⅝"
6'0"	2½"-2¾"

Lower measurements indicate small frame

Higher measurements indicate large frame

330 CALORIES

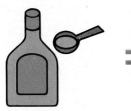

*3 breakfast sausages
(1 ounce each)*

=

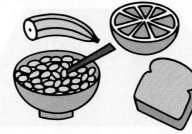

½ grapefruit (3½ ounces)
*1 slice cracked wheat
toast (.9 ounce)*
½ banana (3 ounces)
1 teaspoon sugar
1 cup skim milk   1 cup puffed rice or wheat cereal (1 ounce)

100 CALORIES

*1 tablespoon bottled
French dressing*

=

½ head iceberg lettuce (7½ ounces)
3 large mushrooms (2 ounces)
½ cup carrot (2 ounces)
½ tomato (3 ounces)
4 cucumber slices (2 ounces)   ⅛ cup onion slices (¼ ounce)

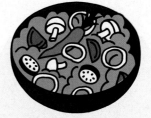

460 CALORIES

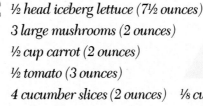

*1 hamburger, ground
chuck (4 ounces)*
1 slice American cheese (1 ounce)
1 hamburger bun (1½ ounces)

=

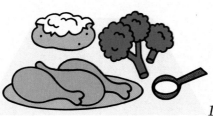

*3 skinless roasted chicken
drumsticks (6 ounces meat)*
1 cup cooked broccoli
1 baked potato (7 ounces)
1 tablespoon plain lowfat yogurt

265 CALORIES

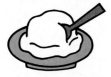

*½ cup premium
vanilla ice cream*

=

1 oatmeal cookie (½ ounce)
1 cup plain lowfat yogurt
1 cup strawberries
1 teaspoon sugar

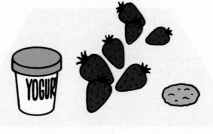

The Calories You Eat

Eliminating dietary calories to the point where you will lose weight does not require eating minuscule amounts of food or counting calories obsessively. The most efficient way of reducing calorie intake is by eating less fat.

By weight, dietary fat contains more than twice the calories of protein and carbohydrates — nine calories per gram compared with four calories per gram of the other two major nutrients. This fact explains why half a cup of peanuts, which contains 34 grams of fat, has nearly four times as many calories as half a cup of kidney beans, which contains only five grams of fat. Likewise, the dishes on the left side of the illustration opposite boast a high fat content that makes them pack a lot of calories in relatively small portions. The dishes on the right, by contrast, are low in fat and so allow you to eat more food for the same number of calories.

In the average American diet, about 40 percent of the total calories consumed are from fat. One major contributor of this fat is red meat. But almost half of dietary fat comes from vegetable oils, shortening and lard, which are used during cooking and baking or added at the table in spreads and dressings. Dairy products and eggs, whose fat content is often highly concentrated, contribute another 15 percent.

Generally, the fat in your diet should supply 30 percent or less of your total calories. Take the first step toward a lowfat diet by assessing the fat content of your current diet. Use the chart on the next two pages — it not only shows calorie values for common foods, but also indicates what percentage of those calories come from fat.

The best way to keep a weight-control diet healthy and relatively satisfying is to replace fatty foods with complex carbohydrates — the starches in grains, cereals, legumes and vegetables. These foods are far lower in calories than an equivalent amount of red meat and contain some vitamins and minerals that meat lacks. You do not have to eliminate meat from your diet, but you should choose the leanest cuts and eat it no more than once a day, in portions of no more than three to four ounces per serving. Or, better yet, eat lean fish or white meat poultry with the skin removed.

Along with cutting back on meat, you should make other low-calorie substitutions to trim your intake of fat and also of refined sugar, another substantial source of calories. Use such dairy products as skim and lowfat milk, and lowfat cheeses and yogurt; avoid fried foods and canned foods packed in oil; eat fruits for desserts and snacks rather than cakes, cookies and other items high in refined sugar as well as fat. The recipes in this book provide an excellent way of incorporating these strategies into your eating plan.

The key to maintaining a low-calorie eating regimen is to take a gradual approach. When you use the recipes and tips in this book steadily to cut a small number of calories from your diet each day, you will soon notice results. Even a daily reduction of only 200 or 300 calories — which you can achieve merely by cutting out the cream in your coffee and the mayonnaise on your sandwich, for example — will allow you to lose a pound in less than two weeks. Changing your diet in small stages keeps you from feeling deprived, which in turn makes it more likely that you will stick with your new eating habits.

A Guide to Calorie Consumption

Food		Portion	Cal.	% Fat
Almonds	slivered	¼ cup	210	83.7
Apple		5 oz	80	11.3
Apple juice		1 cup	120	Trace
Apple pie		4.8 oz slice	345	39.1
Applesauce	sweetened	1 cup	230	Trace
Apricots	dried	¼ cup	83	Trace
Asparagus	cooked	½ cup	45	Trace
Avocado	raw	7.7 oz	370	90
Bacon		2 slices	85	84.7
Bagel	plain	2 oz	165	5.5
Banana		4.25 oz	100	Trace
Bean sprouts	raw	1 cup	35	Trace
Beans	green, cooked	1 cup	30	Trace
Beef	ground, broiled 10% fat	3 oz	185	48.6
	21% fat	3 oz	243	66.7
	rib, broiled lean and fat	3 oz	375	79.2
	lean only	3 oz	208	51.9
	round, broiled lean and fat	3 oz	181	38.2
	lean only	3 oz	165	28
	sirloin, broiled lean and fat	3 oz	330	73.6
	lean only	3 oz	173	31.2
Beef liver	braised	3 oz	195	13.1
Beer		12 fl oz	150	
Beets	cooked	1 cup	55	Trace
Blackberries	raw	1 cup	85	10.6
Blackeyed peas	dried from cooked	1 cup	190	4.7
Blueberries	raw	1 cup	99	Trace
Bouillon	instant	1 cube	5	Trace
Bread	white, enriched	1 slice	75	24
	whole-wheat	1 slice	60	15
Broccoli		1 cup	45	Trace
Brownies	with nuts	2 oz	253	56.9
Brussels sprouts	cooked from raw	1 cup	55	16.4
Butter		1 stick	800	100
Cabbage	raw, shredded	1 cup	15	Trace
	cooked	1 cup	30	Trace
Cake	angel food	2.5 oz	177	Trace
	coffeecake	2.5 oz	221	28.5
	cupcake, chocolate icing	2.5 oz	250	36
	devil's food, choc. icing	2.5 oz	235	30.6
	white, two layer, choc. icing	2.5 oz	250	28.8
	pound cake	2.5 oz	333	54.1
	fruitcake	2.5 oz	254	32.7
Candy	milk chocolate, plain	1 oz	145	55.9
	hard	1 oz	110	Trace
Carrots	grated, raw	1 cup	45	Trace
	cooked	1 cup	50	Trace
Cashew nuts		¼ cup	196	73.5
Cauliflower	raw, chopped	1 cup	31	Trace
	cooked	1 cup	30	Trace
Celery	raw, diced	1 cup	20	Trace
Cereal	wheat flakes, sugared	1 cup	105	Trace
	oatmeal, cooked	1 cup	130	6.9
	40% bran	1 cup	127	8.6
	cornflakes	1 cup	95	Trace
	puffed rice	1 cup	60	Trace
	puffed wheat	1 cup	55	Trace
	shredded wheat	1 biscuit	90	10
	wheat germ	1 tbsp	25	36

Food		Portion	Cal.	% Fat
Cheese	cottage 4% milkfat	8 oz	235	38.3
	2% milkfat	8 oz	200	17.6
	1% milkfat	8 oz	165	10.9
	Cheddar	1 oz	115	70.4
	cream	1 oz	100	90
	mozzarella, part skim	1 oz	80	56.3
	Parmesan, grated	1 tbsp	25	72
	provolone	1 oz	100	72
	ricotta, part skim	9 oz	340	50.3
	Swiss	1 oz	105	68.6
	American	1 oz	105	77.1
Cherries	raw	2.5 oz	45	Trace
Chicken	breast roasted	7 oz	394	36.5
	roasted no skin	7 oz	330	19
	fried no skin	7 oz	374	24.1
	drumstick roasted	3.5 oz	216	45.8
	roasted no skin	3.5 oz	172	10.5
	fried	3.5 oz	268	53.7
	fried no skin	3.5 oz	195	36.9
Colas		12 fl oz	145	Trace
Cookies	chocolate chip	2 oz	286	52.7
	oatmeal with raisins	2 oz	252	32.1
	fig bars	2 oz	200	13.5
	gingersnaps	2 oz	180	20
	macaroons	2 oz	264	45
Corn	cooked from raw	1 ear	70	12.9
	kernels from frozen	1 cup	130	6.9
Crackers	graham	2	55	16.4
	saltines	4	50	18
Cranberry juice cocktail		1 cup	165	Trace
Cucumber slices	peeled	1 oz	5	Trace
Danish pastry		2.3 oz	275	49.1
Dates	chopped	¼ cup	55	Trace
Doughnut	plain cake	2 oz	200	45
Egg	poached	1	80	67.5
	scrambled	1	95	66.3
	fried	1	85	69
	hard-cooked	1	80	67.5
Fish	bluefish, raw	7 oz	234	23.1
	clams, canned	3 oz	45	20
	crabmeat, canned	½ cup	68	19.9
	haddock, raw	7 oz	158	1
	halibut, raw	7 oz	200	9
	oysters, raw	1 cup	165	22.5
	salmon, raw	7 oz	238	45.4
	sardines, canned	3 oz	175	46.3
	scallops, raw	7 oz	162	5.6
	shrimp, raw	3.5 oz	101	9.9
	tuna, canned packed in oil	3.5 oz	207	37.1
	packed in water	3.5 oz	110	7.1
Gin, rum, vodka, whiskey	80 proof	1.5 fl oz	95	
Grape juice		1 cup	165	Trace
Grapefruit	white	½	45	Trace
Grapefruit juice	freshly squeezed	1 cup	95	Trace
	from concentrate	1 cup	100	Trace
Grapes	Thompson seedless	2 oz	35	Trace
Half and half		1 tbsp	20	90
Honey		1 tbsp	65	Trace
Ice cream	hard, vanilla	1 cup	270	47

Food		Portion	Cal.	% Fat
Ice cream	soft, French vanilla	1 cup	377	55
Ice milk	vanilla	1 cup	184	29
Jams and preserves		1 tbsp	55	Trace
Lamb	chop, rib *lean and fat*	3 oz	360	80
	lean only	3 oz	180	45
	leg *lean and fat*	3 oz	235	61.3
	lean only	3 oz	156	34.6
Lemon	raw	2.6 oz	20	Trace
Lemonade	from concentrate	1 cup	105	Trace
Lentils	cooked from raw	1 cup	210	Trace
Lettuce	iceberg	1 cup	5	Trace
Macaroni	cooked	1 cup	155	5.8
Margarine		1 stick	800	100
Mayonnaise		1 tbsp	100	99
Melon	cantaloupe	½	80	Trace
	honeydew	1/10	50	Trace
Milk	whole	1 cup	150	48
	lowfat (2%)	1 cup	120	37.5
	lowfat (1%)	1 cup	100	27
	skim	1 cup	86	Trace
	buttermilk	1 cup	100	18
Milk shake	chocolate	11 oz	368	20
	vanilla	11 oz	350	23.1
Muffin	blueberry	1.5 oz	110	32.7
	bran	1.5 oz	105	34.3
Mushrooms		1 cup	20	Trace
Nondairy creamer	powdered	1 tsp	10	90
Oil	corn	1 tbsp	120	100
	olive	1 tbsp	120	100
	safflower	1 tbsp	120	100
Onions	raw	1 cup	45	Trace
	cooked	1 cup	60	Trace
Orange		4.5 oz	65	Trace
Orange juice	freshly squeezed	1 cup	110	Trace
	from concentrate	1 cup	120	Trace
Pancake	plain	1 oz	60	30
Peach	raw	3.4 oz	40	Trace
Peaches	canned *syrup packed*	1 cup	200	Trace
	water packed	1 cup	75	Trace
Peanut butter		1 tbsp	95	75.8
Peanuts		¼ cup	210	77.1
Pear	Bartlett	5.7 oz	100	9
	canned *syrup packed*	1 cup	195	4.6
Peas	green, raw	1 cup	126	Trace
	green, cooked	1 cup	134	Trace
Peppers	raw	2.5 oz	15	Trace
Pickles	dill	2.3 oz	5	Trace
Pineapple	raw, diced	1 cup	80	Trace
	canned *syrup packed*	1 cup	190	Trace
Pizza	cheese	2 oz slice	145	24.8
Plums	raw	2.4 oz	30	Trace
Popcorn	plain	1 cup	25	Trace
Pork	ham, roasted *lean and fat*	3 oz	245	69.8
	luncheon meat	1 oz slice	65	69.2

Food		Portion	Cal.	% Fat
Pork	chop, loin, broiled *lean and fat*	3 oz	338	74.6
	lean only	3 oz	225	56
	shoulder cut *lean and fat*	3 oz	320	73.1
	lean only	3 oz	184	39.1
Potato	baked with skin	7 oz	216	Trace
	French fried from raw	1.8 oz	135	46.7
Potato chips		¾ oz	115	62.6
Pretzels		2 oz	235	11.5
Prune juice		1 cup	182	Trace
Pudding	chocolate *regular, cooked*	1 cup	320	22.5
	instant	1 cup	325	19.4
Pumpkin pie		4.6 oz	275	49
Raisins		¼ cup	105	Trace
Raspberries	red, raw	1 cup	70	12.9
Rice	white *instant, cooked*	1 cup	180	Trace
	long grain, cooked	1 cup	225	Trace
Roll	frankfurter or hamburger	1.4 oz	120	15
Salad dressing	blue cheese	1 tbsp	75	96
	French	1 tbsp	65	83.1
	Italian	1 tbsp	85	95.3
Sausage	brown and serve	1	70	77.1
	frankfurter	1	170	79.4
	Vienna sausage	1	40	67.5
Sherbet	orange	1 cup	270	13.3
Soup	beef, consommé	1 cup	30	Trace
	split pea	1 cup	145	18.6
	tomato	1 cup	90	30
Spaghetti	enriched, cooked	1 cup	155	5.8
Spinach	raw	1 cup	15	Trace
	cooked from raw	1 cup	40	Trace
Squash	zucchini, cooked	1 cup	30	Trace
	acorn, cooked	1 cup	114	Trace
Strawberries	fresh	1 cup	55	16.4
Sugar	white	1 tbsp	45	Trace
Sunflower seeds		¼ cup	202	75.7
Sweet potato	baked with skin	4 oz	160	5.6
Syrup	chocolate	2 tbsp	125	36
	blackstrap molasses	1 tbsp	45	Trace
Tartar sauce		1 tbsp	75	96
Tomato	raw	4.8 oz	25	Trace
Tomato catsup		1 tbsp	15	Trace
Tomato juice	canned	1 cup	45	Trace
Turkey	roasted *dark meat*	3 oz	175	36
	white meat	3 oz	150	18
Veal	cutlet, braised or broiled	3 oz	185	43.8
	rib, roasted	3 oz	230	54.8
Vinegar	cider	1 tbsp	2	Trace
Waffle	from mix	2.7 oz	205	35.1
Walnuts	chopped	¼ cup	195	88.8
Whipped topping	frozen	1 tbsp	15	60
	pressurized	1 tbsp	10	90
Wine		3.5 fl oz	85	
Yeast	brewer's	1 tbsp	25	Trace
Yogurt	whole milk, *plain*	8 oz	140	45
	skim milk *plain*	8 oz	127	Trace
	lowfat *fruit-flavored*	8 oz	230	3.9

This chart is adapted from *Nutritive Values of Food* compiled by the U.S. Department of Agriculture (USDA) and from *Composition of Foods* (USDA Handbook 8). Caloric and fat content can vary depending upon methods of food processing and analysis.

The figures for fat content indicate the percentage of calories that are derived from fat, not the percentage of fat by weight. ("Trace" means that the percentage of fat is nutritionally negligible.) An effective weight-loss program should limit foods that derive more than 30 percent of their calories from fat.

The Calories You Burn

It is far more difficult to lose weight permanently if you are sedentary than if you are physically active. A number of studies have found that many obese people do not eat significantly more than thinner ones, but the obese are much less active. Similarly, the pound or two of weight that many adults put on yearly when they reach middle age may be due to decreasing physical activity rather than a change in eating patterns. Studies indicate that adults who are physically active throughout their lives maintain a desirable weight.

Researchers have also confirmed that exercise preserves and builds up muscle tissue. Firm muscles not only improve your appearance, but also aid in weight loss because added muscle — unlike body fat — continually burns calories. Moreover, some evidence suggests that vigorous exercise helps to suppress appetite rather than stimulate it, as many people believe.

A crucial part of any weight-loss program, therefore, is adding activities to your daily life that substantially increase calorie expenditure. To do this is not easy: Labor-saving conveniences at work and at home contribute to a sedentary lifestyle. The illustrations opposite show substitutions you can make to replace sedentary routines with more strenuous ones. For example, a brisk 20-minute walk burns up about 120 calories for a 150-pound person. If you did this five days a week for a year rather than ride in a car, you would expend an extra 31,000 calories — equivalent calorically to nearly a nine-pound weight loss.

One group of researchers has estimated that office workers could lose up to 15 pounds a year and homemakers 20 pounds a year by substituting more active behaviors for their normal sedentary routines. The calorie chart on the following two pages will give you an idea of the calories expended for a wide range of daily activities.

The surest way to increase calorie output significantly is with a program of regular exercise. In the following chapters, you will find exercise tips and routines preceding each recipe section. The exercises range from moderate to strenuous levels of exertion, and some of them, particularly the exercises in Chapter Three, are designed to build muscle as you shed weight. To burn off significant amounts of fat, your exercise must be aerobic — meaning that it supplies oxygen to major muscle groups for an extended period. Such exercises, which usually utilize the large muscles of the legs, include running, brisk walking, jumping rope, cycling, aerobic movement, certain calisthentic routines and certain racquet sports. The chart on page 115 will help you choose an exercise and develop a regimen.

As with changing your diet, you are far more likely to make exercise a permanent part of your life if you ease into it gradually. Overexerting yourself can cause you to become fatigued quickly or to injure yourself, and either one increases the likelihood you will give up exercise. If you combine exercising consistently with a reduction in your calorie intake, you will not only take weight off but keep it off.

Getting Active

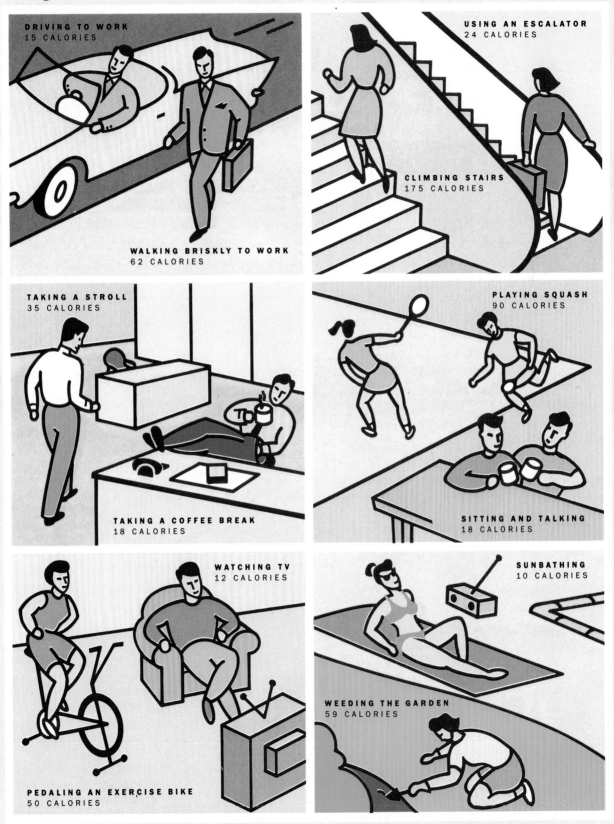

DRIVING TO WORK
15 CALORIES

USING AN ESCALATOR
24 CALORIES

CLIMBING STAIRS
175 CALORIES

WALKING BRISKLY TO WORK
62 CALORIES

TAKING A STROLL
35 CALORIES

PLAYING SQUASH
90 CALORIES

TAKING A COFFEE BREAK
18 CALORIES

SITTING AND TALKING
18 CALORIES

WATCHING TV
12 CALORIES

SUNBATHING
10 CALORIES

WEEDING THE GARDEN
59 CALORIES

PEDALING AN EXERCISE BIKE
50 CALORIES

Calorie counts are for 10 minutes of activity

A Guide to Calorie Expenditure

Activity	Calories burned per minute (by body weight)		
	110 lb	150 lb	190 lb
Ax chopping, fast	14.8	20.2	25.6
Running, level ground, 5.5 min mile	14.4	19.7	24.9
Skin diving, considerable motion	13.8	18.8	23.8
Skiing, cross-country, uphill	13.7	18.6	23.6
Running, 6 min mile	12.6	17.1	21.7
Running, 7 min mile	11.4	15.5	19.6
Boxing	11.1	15.1	19.1
Squash	10.6	14.4	18.3
Running, 8 min mile	10.4	14.1	17.9
Jumping rope, 145 jumps per minute	9.8	13.4	17.0
Judo	9.7	13.3	16.8
Running, 9 min mile	9.6	13.1	16.6
Carrying logs	9.3	12.7	16.0
Racquetball	8.9	12.1	15.3
Jumping rope, 125 jumps per minute	8.8	12.0	15.3
Treading water, fast	8.5	11.6	14.6
Cycling, racing	8.4	11.5	14.6
Swimming, backstroke	8.4	11.5	14.6
Snowshoeing, soft snow	8.3	11.3	14.3
Jumping rope, 80 jumps per minute	8.2	11.2	14.1
Jumping rope, 70 jumps per minute	8.1	11.0	14.0
Swimming, breaststroke, fast	8.1	11.0	14.0
Swimming, crawl, fast	7.8	10.6	13.4
Climbing hill with 44 lb load	7.3	10.0	12.7
Digging trenches	7.2	9.9	12.5
Skiing, cross-country, walking	7.1	9.7	12.3
Marching, rapid	7.1	9.7	12.2
Climbing hill with 22 lb load	7.0	9.5	12.1
Basketball	6.9	9.4	11.9
Boxing, sparring	6.9	9.4	11.9

Activity	Calories burned per minute (by body weight)		
	110 lb	150 lb	190 lb
Forking straw bales	6.9	9.4	11.9
Horseback riding, galloping	6.8	9.3	11.8
Aerobic dance, intense	6.7	9.2	11.6
Running, horizontal, 11.5 min mile	6.7	9.2	11.6
Field hockey	6.7	9.1	11.5
Football	6.6	9.0	11.4
Felling trees	6.6	9.0	11.4
Climbing hills with 9 lb load	6.4	8.8	11.1
Swimming, crawl, slow	6.4	8.7	11.0
Digging	6.3	8.6	10.9
Sawing by hand	6.1	8.3	10.5
Swimming, sidestroke	6.1	8.3	10.5
Climbing hills with no load	6.0	8.2	10.4
Skiing, cross-country, moderate speed	5.9	8.1	10.3
Lawn mowing	5.6	7.6	9.7
Horseback riding, trotting	5.5	7.5	9.5
Planting by hand	5.4	7.4	9.4
Scrubbing floors	5.4	7.4	9.4
Tennis	5.4	7.4	9.4
Shoveling coal	5.4	7.3	9.3
Aerobic dance, medium	5.1	7.0	8.9
Cycling, leisure, 9.5 mph	5.0	6.8	8.6
Skiing, soft snow	4.9	6.7	8.4
Badminton	4.8	6.6	8.4
Weight training, circuit training	4.6	6.3	7.9
Hoeing	4.5	6.2	7.8
Cricket, bowling	4.5	6.1	7.8
Stacking firewood	4.4	6.0	7.6
Weight lifting, free weights	4.3	5.9	7.4
Shoveling grain	4.2	5.8	7.3

Rating Activities

The chart above lists activities and exercises by the number of calories they use up, starting with activities that burn the most. Since almost all energy production by the body uses oxygen, researchers can assess an activity's calorie value by evaluating how much oxygen is used when performing it. You do not use all the oxygen in the air you breathe in, no matter how demanding the activity you are doing, and therefore your exhaled air contains some oxygen. To determine the amount of oxygen an activity requires, researchers collect a subject's exhaled air in a rubber bag during an activity and then compare the amount of oxygen in this exhaled air with the amount of oxygen in the ambient air. The difference in the percentages of ox-

Activity	Calories burned per minute (by body weight)			Activity	Calories burned per minute (by body weight)		
	110 lb	150 lb	190 lb		110 lb	150 lb	190 lb
Golf	4.2	5.8	7.3	Cooking	2.4	3.3	4.1
Cricket, batting	4.1	5.6	7.2	Wallpapering	2.4	3.3	4.1
Walking, normal pace, fields and hills	4.1	5.6	7.1	Violin playing, sitting	2.2	3.1	3.9
Walking, normal pace, grass	4.0	5.5	7.0	Sewing by machine	2.2	3.1	3.9
Walking, normal pace, asphalt road	4.0	5.4	6.9	Canoeing	2.2	3.0	3.8
Plastering	3.9	5.3	6.7	Billiards	2.1	2.9	3.6
House painting, exteriors	3.8	5.2	6.6	Horseback riding, walking	2.0	2.8	3.5
Walking, normal pace, plowed field	3.8	5.2	6.6	Cello playing, sitting	2.0	2.8	3.5
Sawing, power	3.7	5.1	6.5	Driving harvester	2.0	2.7	3.4
Weeding	3.6	4.9	6.2	Piano playing, sitting	2.0	2.7	3.4
Table tennis	3.4	4.6	5.9	Conducting music	1.9	2.7	3.4
Gymnastics	3.3	4.5	5.7	Bookbinding	1.9	2.6	3.3
Playing drums, sitting	3.3	4.5	5.7	Driving tractor	1.8	2.5	3.2
Archery	3.2	4.4	5.6	Drawing, standing	1.8	2.4	3.1
Cycling, 5.5 mph	3.2	4.4	5.5	Flute playing, sitting	1.7	2.4	3.0
Scraping paint	3.1	4.3	5.4	Accordion playing, sitting	1.6	2.2	2.8
Fishing	3.1	4.2	5.3	Woodwind playing, sitting	1.6	2.2	2.8
Food shopping	3.1	4.2	5.3	Sewing by hand	1.6	2.2	2.8
Mopping floors	3.1	4.2	5.3	Trumpet playing, standing	1.5	2.1	2.7
Treading water, normal	3.1	4.2	5.3	Typing, manual	1.5	2.1	2.7
Croquet	2.9	4.0	5.1	Horn playing, sitting	1.4	2.0	2.5
Cleaning	2.9	3.9	5.0	Writing, sitting	1.4	2.0	2.5
Window cleaning	2.9	3.9	5.0	Standing still	1.3	1.8	2.3
Milking cows by hand	2.7	3.7	4.7	Typing, electric	1.3	1.8	2.3
Raking	2.7	3.7	4.7	Card playing	1.2	1.7	2.2
Organ playing, sitting	2.6	3.6	4.6	Eating, sitting	1.1	1.6	2.0
Carpentry	2.6	3.5	4.5	Milking cows by machine	1.1	1.6	2.0
Welding	2.6	3.5	4.5	Knitting	1.1	1.5	1.9
Dancing, ballroom	2.5	3.5	4.4	Lying still	1.1	1.5	1.9
Volleyball	2.5	3.4	4.3	Sitting still	1.0	1.4	1.8

ygen allows researchers to calculate how many calories were expended.

For any activity, however, the energy cost is affected by a multitude of factors that varies from person to person. For example, as the chart indicates, the heavier you are, the more calories you will burn performing many activities. This is because the added pounds contribute to the effort of any movement.

Your level of conditioning, the temperature and humidity of the air and how efficiently you perform an activity also affect calorie expenditure.

Although the values are approximate rather than precise measurements, you can use this chart to estimate the number of calories you burn during exertion. Choosing the more energetic activities will aid you in reducing your weight.

Planning Your Meals

When you take the responsibility for planning your own meals, rather than following a set diet, you can choose foods that please your palate and satisfy your hunger while meeting your calorie limitations and fulfilling your nutritional needs. Although you should be aware of the calorie content of foods, you do not have to count every calorie in order to lose weight. Just keep in mind three principles: Eat foods that are low in fat and high in complex carbohydrates, eat modest portions and eat a variety of foods.

The menus on these two pages — intended as examples, not blueprints — show you how to apply these principles. Each menu totals 1,500-1,600 calories daily, which nutritionists consider the minimum for most people on a weight-loss program that includes exercise.

These menus combine recipes from this book with other foods to lend variety to the meals and to meet nutritional requirements; however, any eating plan that restricts your calories also limits your intake of vitamins and minerals. On page 38, you will find a set of guidelines to ensure that your weight-loss program stays nutritionally balanced.

Weekday breakfasts have to be fast: Make a batch of whole-grain muffins and freeze them individually. In the morning, heat one in the toaster. For snacks at work, keep some lowfat crackers in your desk so that you can avoid vending-machine fare or other readily available high-calorie foods. Skim or lowfat milk, a good source of calcium and B vitamins, can be added to meals or snacks.

For lunch, a salad you make the night before can be taken to work in an insulated container. At afternoon break time, fill up on vegetables with a low-calorie spread.

After work, it takes just minutes to prepare a salad and stir-fry precooked chicken and broccoli (using a combination of chicken stock and oil to save calories).

WEEKDAY

	Calories
Breakfast	
Cornmeal-Cheese English Muffin with herbed ricotta spread (page 54)	367
Coffee or tea (optional)	
Mid-morning snack	
6 Rye-Cheese Crackers (page 71)	85
1/2 cup lowfat milk (2%)	60
Lunch	
Tampa Bay Halibut Salad (page 92)	305
1/2 cup lowfat milk (2%)	60
Medium-size peach	40
Mid-afternoon snack	
White Bean-Chèvre Spread (page 106)	192
Dinner	
Large spinach-mushroom salad with 3 tablespoons yogurt-orange juice dressing	80
3 ounces poached chicken breast and 4 ounces blanched broccoli, stir-fried with scallions and ginger in a nonstick skillet using 1 teaspoon oil and 2 tablespoons chicken stock; served with 1/2 cup cooked rice	340
total	1,529

SPECIAL OCCASION

	Calories
Breakfast	
1 cup (1 ounce) vitamin-mineral fortified cereal	100
1/2 cup lowfat milk (2%)	60
1/2 cup sliced strawberries	28
Mid-morning snack	
1/2 cup lowfat vanilla yogurt	100
Coffee or tea (optional)	
Lunch	
Curried Vegetable Soup (page 91)	265
1/2 cup lowfat milk (2%)	60
Mid-afternoon snack	
1/2 cup lowfat vanilla yogurt	100
Dinner (restaurant)	
Tossed salad of leaf lettuce, Romaine, cucumber and tomatoes; request oil and vinegar on the side and use no more than 2 teaspoons of oil	105
6 ounces lean roast leg of lamb	
1/2 cup herbed rice	
1/2 cup steamed asparagus	
1 teaspoon butter	450
4 ounces red wine	85
Small slice chocolate layer cake	230
total	1,583

Although you should try to focus on the nonfood aspects of celebrations, advance planning permits you to indulge in certain foods you would otherwise avoid.

Eating fewer calories earlier in the day allows you to "bank" some calories for a glass of wine and/or a dessert at dinner. Just be sure that your breakfast, lunch and snack foods supply the required vitamins and minerals.

The restaurant dinner here begins with a salad—a good start because it takes the edge off your appetite. Eat slowly, and do not feel obliged to finish oversized restaurant portions. Try to stop when you are almost full: You can then go ahead and enjoy a modest dessert.

WEEKEND

	Calories
Pre-exercise snack	
Strawberry-Orange Milk Shake (page 52)	124
Pineapple-Oatmeal Muffin (page 63)	187
Breakfast	
Gingerbread Brown-Rice Pancakes (page 64)	245
Lunch	
Tomato filled with 2 ounces water-packed tuna, 2 tablespoons lowfat yogurt, 2 tablespoons chopped celery; served on 1/2 cup spinach leaves	115
1 cup lowfat milk (2%)	120
10 dried apricot halves	83
Mid-afternoon snack	
Fruit-Bowl Drink (page 104)	101
Dinner	
Greek Salad (page 121)	170
Lentil Minestrone (page 128)	286
Lime Bavarian (page 100)	141
total	1,572

On weekends, when you have extra time, you may plan a longer workout than you can fit in during the week.

You may want a snack before you exercise; if so, choose the shake or the muffin —or both. After your workout, enjoy a leisurely breakfast of pancakes.

Lunch is easy and low in calories but provides substantial protein, calcium and iron. The fruit drink refreshes you during the afternoon and contains plenty of vitamins A and C.

You probably have more time to cook on weekends, so this dinner is a bit more elaborate than the usual weekday meal. A large salad and a hearty soup are followed by a dessert you can make in the afternoon, or the night before, and chill until dinnertime.

Low-calorie Cooking

The recipes in this volume are designed to fit a menu plan of 1,500-1,600 calories per day: 300-400 calories contained in each of three meals, and about 300-400 calories divided between two snacks. The recipes were created to provide a variety of flavors and textures and to include dishes from a range of cuisines. The exam-

ple below, a main-dish salad, highlights some of the ways these recipes provide generous amounts of food while limiting calories through the careful choice of ingredients and the use of cooking techniques that require little or no fat. You can use these principles in choosing recipes from other sources to suit a low-calorie, lowfat diet.

A The recipe headnote highlights a particularly important nutrient or a low-calorie ingredient that is contained in the recipe.

B These recipes include a minimal amount of meat—enough for good nutrition, but not so much as to make the dishes overly high in fat and protein. In this recipe, ½ pound of chicken for four servings is supplemented with a large amount of high-carbohydrate vegetables. Removing the chicken skin before cooking is an example of a technique that cuts fat content—here, by about 50 percent.

C Wherever possible, the use of oil in these recipes is limited, since oils are 100 percent fat. In this case, chicken stock substitutes as the main basis for the salad dressing, which keeps the oil and fat content down.

D Many conventional recipes depend on high-fat ingredients to provide flavor. In the recipes in this book, herbs are used to heighten flavor without adding calories.

E Throughout the book, greens are used in generous amounts: They are very filling because of their high fiber content but low in calories. (All the vegetables in one serving of this dish add up to just 66 calories.)

F The ingredients for these recipes are chosen for their nutritional content as well as for their taste and low calories. The mango used here has only 135 calories, but supplies more than the RDA of vitamins A and C. It also contains generous amounts of potassium and niacin.

G Techniques like poaching, which keeps chicken and fish moist and tender, are used instead of methods like frying, which adds fat.

H Prepare your greens as close as possible to serving time to preserve taste and nutrients.

I The calorie counts for main dishes in this book are below 400; for snacks, the average serving does not exceed 200 calories.

J The percentages in the nutrition charts refer to carbohydrates, protein and fat as ratios of the total calorie count, not of the weight of the ingredients (which is given in grams). This dish, like the others in this book, conforms to American Heart Association guidelines for high-carbohydrate/lowfat eating (see page 38).

K The calcium and iron listings are designed to help you calculate your intake of these two important minerals. The chart on page 39 will help you identify sources for calcium and iron to ensure that you get enough.

L The recipes in this book keep salt to a minimum and limit high-sodium ingredients.

GREEN SALAD WITH CHICKEN AND MANGOES

(A) *Niacin is found in fatty foods such as beef and peanuts, but you can get half your daily requirement of niacin from the chicken and mangoes in this salad.*

(B) 1/2 pound boneless, skinless
chicken breast
1/2 cup low-sodium chicken stock
(C) 1/4 cup lemon juice
2 tablespoons olive oil
(D) 1 teaspoon finely chopped fresh
tarragon, or 1/4 teaspoon dried
tarragon, crumbled

1/4 teaspoon salt
1/4 teaspoon black pepper
2 heads Romaine lettuce
2 bunches watercress
(E) 2 cups diced red bell peppers
1 cup shredded red cabbage
1 cup finely chopped scallions
4 mangoes, peeled and diced (F)

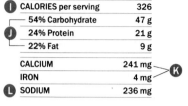

(I) CALORIES per serving	326	
⌐ 54% Carbohydrate	47 g	
(J) 24% Protein	21 g	
└ 22% Fat	9 g	
CALCIUM	241 mg	(K)
IRON	4 mg	
(L) SODIUM	236 mg	

(G) Place the chicken in a small saucepan, add cold water to cover and bring to a boil over medium-high heat. Reduce the heat so that the water simmers and poach the chicken for 5 minutes, or just until cooked through; transfer it to a plate and set aside to cool to room temperature.

For the dressing, in a small bowl whisk together the stock, lemon juice, oil, tarragon, salt and pepper; set aside. Wash the Romaine and watercress. Tear the Romaine into bite-size pieces, trim the watercress and combine the greens (H) in a large bowl. Add the cabbage and scallions, and toss well.

Cut the chicken diagonally into thin slices. Whisk the dressing briefly to reblend it. Add the chicken, mangoes and dressing to the salad and toss gently. Divide the salad among 4 plates and serve.   Makes 4 servings

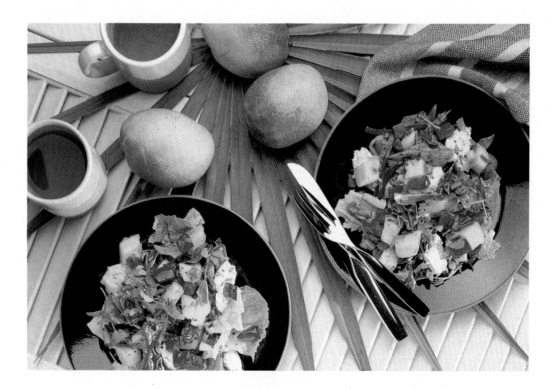

Nutritional Guidelines

The nutrition charts that accompany the recipes in this book include the number of calories per serving, the number of grams of fat, carbohydrate and protein in a serving, and the percentage of calories derived from each of these nutrients. The charts also provide the amount of calcium, iron and sodium per serving. Although the number of calories taken in and expended is what actually determines whether you will gain or lose weight, the fat, carbohydrate and protein makeup of your diet is most important to your health. The National Institutes of Health recommends a diet in which no more than 30 percent of the calories come from fat, 55 to 60 percent come from carbohydrates and no more than 15 percent come from protein. A gram of fat equals nine calories, while a gram of protein or carbohydrate equals four calories; therefore, if you eat 1,500 calories a day, you should consume approximately 50 grams of fat, 200 grams of carbohydrate and no more than 55 grams of protein daily.

◆ The fats you consume should be mainly monounsaturated and polyunsaturated fats, such as those found in most vegetable oils. The saturated fat found in meat, high-fat dairy products, palm oil and coconut oil is associated with the formation of cholesterol in the blood, and elevated blood cholesterol levels play a significant role in heart disease.

◆ Most of the carbohydrates you eat should be complex (such as those found in grains, beans and starchy vegetables) rather than simple (the sugars common in highly processed foods). Fruits contain fructose, a simple carbohydrate, but they also contain vitamins, minerals and fiber.

◆ Look to lowfat protein sources: Substitute chicken or fish for red meat and use vegetable protein sources such as grain products and beans. The average American diet supplies more protein than most people require, so if you eat less meat, you will probably not be lacking for protein.

◆ A low-calorie diet may reduce your intake of four nutrients — calcium, iron, niacin and thiamine — that are essential to good health, as explained below. The box opposite lists low-calorie sources for these nutrients and gives the recommended dietary allowance, or RDA, for each. The RDA refers to the recommended level of intake for nutrients as determined by the Food and Nutrition Board of the National Research Council of the National Academy of Sciences. The recommended levels are those adequate "to meet the known nutritional needs of practically all healthy persons."

◆ Calcium deficiency may result in osteoporosis, or bone shrinking and weakening, in the elderly. Among those most at risk for this disease are women who repeatedly adopt low-calorie, lowfat diets that lack many of the best calcium sources. Calcium deficiency is also linked with periodontal disease and may contribute to high blood pressure. Two of the best sources of calcium are lowfat and skim milk. However, milk products are not the only source of calcium, as the box opposite shows.

◆ Iron is vital to oxygen transport within the body. Women who exercise strenuously and who diet are particularly at risk of iron deficiency. If you reduce your intake of red meat, the best natural source of dietary iron, try to eat some of the foods listed on the opposite page. The iron in vegetables, fruits, grains and beans can be better absorbed by the body when these foods are eaten with small amounts of animal protein and foods that contain vitamin C (such as citrus fruits or tomatoes).

◆ Niacin and thiamine may be a problem for those on weight-loss diets, since these two B vitamins are present mainly in fatty foods like meat and nuts. Both vitamins play a vital role in releasing energy from the food you eat and in regulating brain and nerve function.

◆ Most adults should restrict sodium intake to 1,000 milligrams per 1,000 calories consumed, according to the American Heart Association. One way to keep sodium consumption in check is to avoid adding table salt to food.

FOUR KEY NUTRIENTS

The foods listed below are good sources of the important vitamins and minerals covered in the guidelines on the opposite page. Many of them are included in the recipes in this book and may already be part of your diet. If they are not, incorporating them in your meals will help ensure adequate nutrition.

CALCIUM	mg	calories
RDA: Women 1200 mg; men 800 mg		
Nonfat yogurt, *1 cup*	451	127
Sardines, canned, with bones, *3 ounces*	371	175
Skim milk, *1 cup*	302	86
Cheddar cheese, *1 ounce*	204	115
Bok choy, *1 cup cooked*	158	20
Tofu, *4 ounces*	145	82
Molasses, blackstrap, *1 tablespoon*	140	43
Kale, *1 cup cooked*	94	42
Cottage cheese, lowfat (2%), *½ cup*	78	100

Even if you cut down on some dairy products to reduce fat intake, you can still get a good supply of calcium from lowfat dairy products and green vegetables.

IRON	mg	calories
RDA:Women 18 mg; men 10 mg		
Vitamin-mineral fortified breakfast cereal, *1 ounce*	18.0	100
Liver, beef, braised, *3 ounces*	5.8	195
Molasses, blackstrap, *1 tablespoon*	3.3	43
Prune juice, *1 cup*	3.0	182
Potato, baked, with skin, *7 ounces*	2.7	216
Navy beans, *½ cup cooked*	2.6	112
Apricots, dried, *10 halves*	1.7	83
Shrimp, raw, *3½ ounces*	1.8	101
Broccoli, *1 cup cooked*	1.8	45

Liver, one of the best iron sources, should not be eaten often because it is high in fat and cholesterol. The other foods listed are low in fat and most have no cholesterol.

THIAMINE	mg	calories
RDA: Women 1 mg; men 1.4 mg		
Brewer's yeast, *1 tablespoon*	1.25	25
Pork, lean center loin, broiled, *3 ounces*	.97	196
40% bran cereal, *1 cup*	.51	127
Wheat germ, toasted, *¼ cup*	.47	100
Green peas, *¾ cup cooked*	.31	100
Oatmeal, fortified instant, *1 packet*	.30	101
Peanuts, raw, skinless, *1 ounce*	.28	161
Asparagus, *1 cup cooked*	.18	45

Thiamine, a B vitamin, must be constantly replenished because the body does not store it effectively. Fortified cereals, whole grains and legumes are lowfat sources.

NIACIN	mg	calories
RDA: Women 13 mg; men 18 mg		
Chicken breast, skinless, roasted, *3 ounces*	11.7	140
Tuna, water-packed, *3 ounces*	10.0	95
Halibut, raw, *3½ ounces*	8.3	100
Round steak, lean only, broiled, *3 ounces*	5.1	165
Oysters, *1 cup*	3.1	165
Lima beans, *½ cup cooked*	.9	104

Peanut butter, one of the best niacin sources, is high in fat. Lean meat, poultry, fish, shellfish and legumes are lower in fat and provide good amounts of niacin.

Keeping Track

Studies of people who change their eating habits show that keeping a diary is an important tool for successful weight control. Immediately writing down what you eat whenever you eat ensures your awareness of your food intake. Likewise, chronicling your exercise demonstrates how active you are.

When examined at the end of a week or more, the daily eating and exercise diary provides an accurate picture of your behavior patterns as well. You can compile your own diary by photocopying the opposite page, or you can create your own.

Start your diary at least one week before you plan to change your eating and exercise habits. During that first week, eat and exercise as usual. Do not eliminate any high-calorie foods that you ordinarily consume, and do not allow yourself an overly large portion of fattening dishes as a last indulgence before you cut calories. Also, stick to your normal exercise regimen. Your diary for this period should give an accurate picture of your typical meals, snacks and activities. When you compare your normal pattern to your new habits, you can begin to assess their impact on your weight.

In the diet section of your diary, along with the foods you consume, make a note of where you eat, the distractions that are present and the mood you are in. All these observations are aids for identifying and eventually changing habitual patterns that contribute to overeating.

After a week, examine your diary for habits that contribute to your excess weight. Note the times and places that you are most likely to eat fattening snack foods.

Another important item worth analyzing is what other activities you perform while you eat. Eating on the run or in your car and nibbling while you are preparing a meal are common habits to avoid when you are cutting calories from your diet.

If you find that you cannot resist buying high-fat snacks in the supermarket, you can schedule your shopping trips for after mealtime, when you feel full. Or, if you find that you eat to offset depression at a certain hour of the day or day of the week, you can plan another kind of mood-elevating activity, such as exercise, for that time period.

Then, after you have begun a low-calorie diet, use your diary to chart your progress. Are there problem areas in your daily diet that are particularly hard to change? Instead of abstaining from snacks at work, for example try substituting low-calorie foods like raw vegetables. You will probably find that switching to alternative foods is easier than eliminating the habit entirely.

An advantage to keeping a diary while you are cutting calories is that the very act of writing down what you eat may act as a deterrent to overeating. You may be better able to resist a tempting, fattening food if you know your diary will act as a silent witness.

Once you reach your desired weight, continue your diary for at least a few weeks to make sure that you retain your new eating habits. At this stage of your weight program, the diary will act as a reinforcement of your new habits.

· *Daily Eating and Exercise Diary* ·

DATE

TIME	FOOD	AMOUNT	PLACE	DISTRACTIONS	MOOD

EXERCISE	TIME	PLACE	DURATION	MOOD

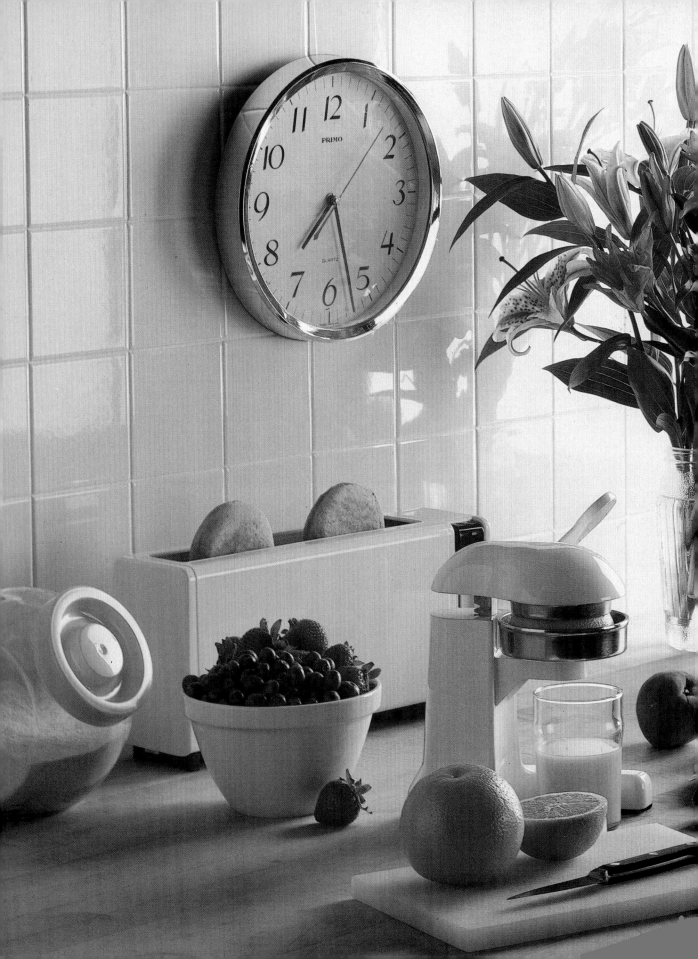

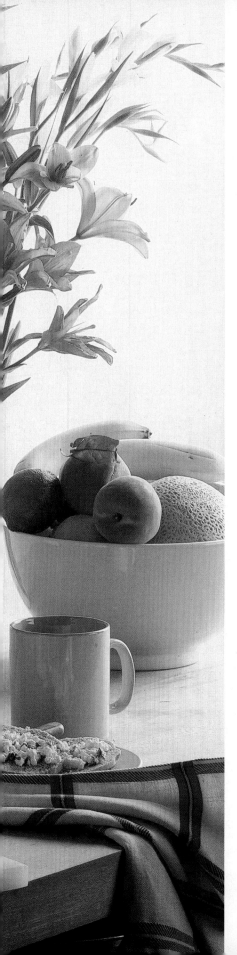

CHAPTER TWO

Breakfast

A filling start for the day

Ｉf you are trying to lose weight, you may be skimping on breakfast or skipping it altogether. Either out of concern for their weight or because they are rushed in the morning, millions of Americans — one out of every four adults — forgo breakfast most or all the time. And surveys show that breakfast is more likely to be skipped than lunch or dinner. In fact, there is no evidence to suggest that skipping breakfast helps produce weight loss; in fact, a case can be made that eating early in the day is one of the best steps you can take toward that goal.

As a means of controlling calories, the chief advantage of starting the day with a good breakfast is that it helps keep you from overeating later. A national food-consumption survey by the U.S. Department of Agriculture found that breakfast skippers were more likely to snack later and to consume snacks higher in calories than breakfast eaters.

The person who eats little or no breakfast may eat an unusually large lunch, or else skimp on lunch, snack through the afternoon and then eat a great deal at dinner. Yet for people concerned about their weight, evening may not be the best time to consume the bulk of their calories. In several recent studies, two groups of subjects were fed only once a day, either at breakfast or at dinner. Both groups consumed the same number of calories. Most of the subjects lost more weight on the morning-meal regimen. Although the studies involved only a handful of subjects, the research suggests that the body may burn calories eaten in the morning more readily than those eaten at night.

Of course, what you eat for this meal is as important as whether you eat it. Some traditional breakfast foods, such as eggs, bacon, sausage, cream, butter, whole milk and cream cheese, are very high in fat and cholesterol. Even a modest breakfast comprised of these foods can add up to 800 calories. An increasingly popular form of breakfast — the breakfast sandwich served in fast-food restaurants — is likewise high in calories and fat: In a survey of fast-food breakfast dishes, several of the sandwiches containing eggs and meat had more than 500 calories each, with 60 percent or more of the calories coming from fat.

A breakfast made up mainly of high-fat foods not only inhibits weight loss, but is also nutritionally unsound: The saturated fat in eggs, meat and dairy products tends to raise cholesterol levels, and fatty foods are generally low in the vitamins and minerals that make up a healthy diet, particularly vitamin C and calcium. Skipping breakfast avoids fat, but it also deprives you of nutrients. Nor is your body properly fueled on a meal of coffee and toast.

There are many strategies you can adopt to make breakfasts that are nourishing and also help you control your weight. First, you can choose lowfat versions of traditional breakfast foods. For example, instead of whole milk, which has 150 calories per cup, use skim milk, which has only 86. Use egg whites rather than whole eggs: All the fat and cholesterol are in the yolk. Egg whites are an excellent source of protein and they help bind ingredients, as in the Gingerbread-Brown Rice Pancakes on page 64. An alternative to butter is lowfat cheese, such as the ricotta used on the Cornmeal-Cheese English Muffins on page 54. You can avoid excessive sugar at breakfast by trying homemade fruit juices and sauces, which make nutritious low-calorie sweeteners — for example, as a topping for the French Toast Fingers on page 50.

Second, expand your definition of what is suitable as a breakfast dish. There is no reason why vegetables and legumes, which are relatively low in calories and high in fiber and complex carbohydrates, cannot be eaten in the morning — and these foods have the benefit of filling you up, as do less familiar whole grains like bulgur. A wide variety of foods are explored in many of the recipes that follow, like the Baked Sweet Potato Doughnuts on page 56, Tortillas Rancheras, filled with vegetables and beans, on page 52 and Oatmeal-Bulgur Cereal with Tangerines on page 65.

Third, some advance planning can simplify your morning routine

Choosing a Cereal

Ready-to-eat cereals are not only convenient, but can offer a filling low-calorie breakfast. Studies show that people who eat cereal for breakfast generally consume less fat and fewer calories than those who rely on other conventional breakfast foods. Unfortunately, some popular cereals are loaded with refined sugar and fat. The following suggestions will help you choose a packaged cereal that gives you the most nutritive value for your calories:

◆ Study the cereal box label. In general, the shorter the list of ingredients, the more nutritious the cereal. Ideally, a whole grain should be listed first: This means it is the main component. One ounce of cereal, the amount usually given as one serving, can range from 50 to 130 calories. Most of these calories are from carbohydrates, but be sure they are from the complex variety — grains — rather than from simple sugars. In some popular cereals, refined sweeteners make up 40 to 60 percent of the weight, the equivalent of four heaping teaspoons of sugar in one ounce of cereal. The ratio (in grams) of total carbohydrates to protein should be about 8 to 1. If the ratio is greater, the cereal probably provides too much refined sugar.

◆ Most ready-to-eat cereals are relatively low in fat, with one to three grams per ounce. But granola cereals tend to have much more fat than other types — at least four grams per ounce, as much as a pat and a half of butter. Most of this fat may be highly saturated palm oil or coconut oil, both of which can contribute to raised cholesterol levels. You are better off eating homemade granola, prepared with as little oil as possible.

◆ Cereals can be a good source of dietary fiber, one of the best food components to help control weight *(pages 46-47)*. High-fiber cereals contain up to 13 grams of fiber per serving.

so that you have time to eat and enjoy breakfast. Bake breads or muffins in advance or, for recipes with short cooking times, measure out and prepare the ingredients the night before.

If you are one of those people who have no appetite until they have been up for an hour or two — and you have to be at work fairly early — take something nourishing with you when you leave home in the morning. If you do eat a complete breakfast but still get hungry before lunchtime, keep your hunger at bay with one of the light, nutritious snacks on pages 70-73. An essential component of a weight-loss regimen is for you to feel relatively full until it is time for your next meal. You can achieve that feeling with far fewer calories than you might expect.

Finally, when you have no time or inclination to cook, you can put together a nutritious, low-calorie quick breakfast. Couscous-Currant Cereal on page 52 takes only minutes to make, as do the two fruit milk shakes on pages 52 and 64. Ready-to-eat cereals with fruit and lowfat milk also provide quick yet satisfying meals as long as you choose cereals with an eye for sound nutrition *(see box above)*.

Feeling Full

There is no mystery as to why a traditional breakfast of eggs, bacon and buttered toast fills you up. Such a meal is high in fat, and fat slows the process of food emptying from your stomach, making you feel full. But you can achieve the same result without eating fatty foods. People who regularly consume foods high in dietary fiber find it easier to keep their weight down since fiber is filling but does not add calories.

Fiber is the part of plants that passes through your system undigested after you eat. The bran in whole-grain breads and cereals is probably the most familiar form of fiber, but — as the chart opposite shows — fruits, vegetables, oats, nuts and legumes like kidney beans and lentils are also high-fiber foods.

One characteristic of cellulose, the fiber most commonly found in whole grains, is that it absorbs water, which helps contribute to a feeling of fullness. In addition, fiber expands quickly in the stomach and small intestine so that you feel full sooner, and the sensation of fullness, or satiety, lasts relatively long. The texture of many high-fiber foods can also make them take longer to chew than foods high in fat, and this helps slow you down while eating. Not only do fibrous foods compare favorably with fatty foods in terms of fewer calories, but they also tend to be much better sources of vitamin A and the mineral potassium.

The American Dietetic Association recommends that adults consume 25 to 35 grams of dietary fiber daily. Most Americans consume only five to 10 grams daily. If you should increase your fiber intake, do so gradually; otherwise, you may irritate the lining of your intestines or suffer gas or diarrhea. Here are some suggestions for getting more fiber into your diet.

● Eat a variety of foods. This will help ensure that you get the benefits of various forms of fiber. By aiding the passage of food through the large intestine, insoluble fibers such as cellulose not only fill you up, but may also help prevent a range of intestinal disorders, from constipation to colon cancer. Water-soluble fibers, which are found mainly in fruits, vegetables, and grains like barley and oats, do less to help the passsage of food, but they appear to lower blood cholesterol.

● Eat raw fruits and vegetables as a mid morning snack. Fruit and vegetables like apples, carrots and broccoli are rich in fiber, but they should be eaten raw — boiling, peeling and processing tend to reduce the fiber content of these foods.

● Drink liquids when you eat high-fiber foods. Water and other fluids help you feel full by taking up space in your stomach. And when consumed with sufficient fluids, fiber helps regulate bowel function.

● Spread out your fiber intake. Breakfast is an excellent time to eat high-fiber foods, particularly breakfast cereals. Getting all your fiber at one sitting, however, may increase the chance of unpleasant side effects. As a general rule, you should have foods containing both water-soluble and water-insoluble fiber at every meal.

HIGH-FIBER FOODS

Food	Serving	Dietary Fiber (grams)
WHOLE BRAN CEREAL	1/2 cup	12.9
KIDNEY BEANS, COOKED	1/2 cup	7.3
RAISINS	1/2 cup	6.2
PEAR WITH SKIN	1 large	6.2
NAVY BEANS, COOKED	1/2 cup	6.0
SPAGHETTI, WHOLE-WHEAT	1 cup	3.9
LENTILS, COOKED	1/2 cup	3.7
PEAS, COOKED	1/2 cup	3.6
APPLE WITH SKIN	1 medium	3.5
SWEET POTATO, COOKED	1 medium	3.4
WHEAT GERM	1/4 cup	3.4
ALMONDS	1/4 cup	3.3
RASPBERRIES	1/2 cup	3.1
PRUNES	3	3.0
PARSNIPS, COOKED	1/2 cup	2.7
RAISIN BRAN CEREAL	1/2 cup	2.7
ORANGE	1 medium	2.6
POTATO WITH SKIN, COOKED	1 medium	2.5
BANANA	1 medium	2.4
BRUSSELS SPROUTS, COOKED	1/2 cup	2.3
CARROTS, COOKED	1/2 cup	2.3
BROCCOLI, COOKED	1/2 cup	2.2
SPINACH, COOKED	1/2 cup	2.1
BLUEBERRIES	1/2 cup	2.0
DATES	3	1.9
WHEAT, SHREDDED	1/2 cup	1.9
PEACH WITH SKIN	1 medium	1.9
ZUCCHINI, COOKED	1/2 cup	1.8
GREEN BEANS, COOKED	1/2 cup	1.6
TURNIPS, COOKED	1/2 cup	1.6
BEAN SPROUTS, RAW	1/2 cup	1.5
APRICOTS, DRIED	5 halves	1.4
BREAD, WHOLE-WHEAT	1 slice	1.4
CABBAGE, COOKED	1/2 cup	1.4
SUMMER SQUASH, COOKED	1/2 cup	1.4
CHERRIES	10	1.2
CELERY, RAW	1/2 cup	1.1
SPAGHETTI, REGULAR	1 cup	1.1
PINEAPPLE	1/2 cup	1.1
ASPARAGUS, COOKED	1/2 cup	1.0
BREAD, CRACKED-WHEAT	1 slice	1.0
BROWN RICE, COOKED	1/2 cup	1.0
CANTALOUPE	1/4 melon	1.0
LETTUCE, RAW	1 cup	0.9

Continuous Calisthenics

A calisthenics routine at the start of the day provides an excellent nonstressful way to raise your metabolism and your body temperature. Calisthenics can also burn 100 to 200 calories or more in less than half an hour if performed vigorously.

The exercises on this and the opposite page are meant to follow one another as a continuous series. Perform each exercise for several minutes so that the routine adds up to a 20-minute workout.

Jogging in place is an excellent way to warm up and cool down, since you can easily regulate its intensity. Before you begin your routine, jog in place for three to five minutes, gradually increasing the intensity until you break a light sweat. After you have completed the calisthenics routine, jog in place again to perform a five-minute cool-down.

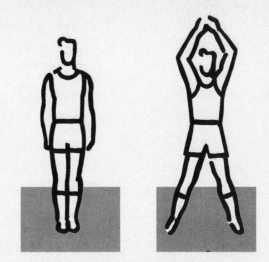

1. To perform jumping jacks, stand with your feet together and your hands at your sides. Hop so that your feet land apart and your hands touch above your head.

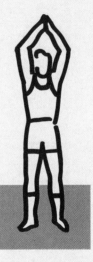

2. Perform a series of heel touches. First, stand with your feet apart and your hands touching. Squat down and touch your ankles. Return to the standing position and repeat.

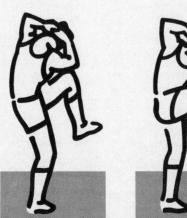

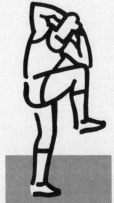

3. Interlace your fingers behind your head and lift your left knee to touch it with your right elbow. Alternate right knee and left elbow and back again.

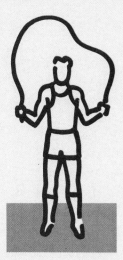

4. Jump rope with a two-footed hop, landing on the balls of your feet with your knees slightly bent. Jump no more than an inch in the air to avoid the risk of injury.

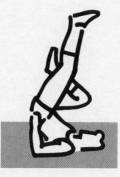

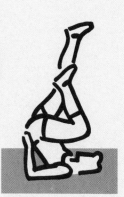

5. Lie on your back, lift your feet toward the ceiling and support your pelvis with your hands. Alternately kick up and down as if you were pedaling a bicycle.

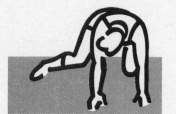

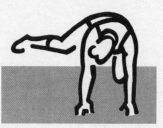

6. Kneel on all fours and extend one foot out to the side *(far left)*. Keep your knee slightly flexed and raise your leg. Then repeat for the opposite leg.

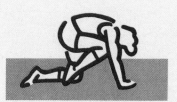

7. Perform hip and leg extensions by kneeling on all fours and drawing your right knee to your chin. Swing your right leg out and up, then bring it back to your chin. Swing one leg, then the other.

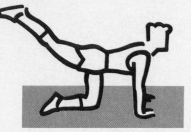

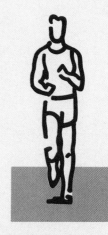

8. Run in place and gradually reduce your exercise intensity to cool down. Spend at least three to five minutes cooling down.

49

FRENCH TOAST FINGERS WITH APPLE PUREE

A warm, unsweetened fruit sauce tops this whole-wheat French toast.

CALORIES per serving	350
59% Carbohydrate	55 g
13% Protein	12 g
28% Fat	11 g
CALCIUM	92 mg
IRON	3 mg
SODIUM	318 mg

4 Granny Smith apples, peeled, cored and thinly sliced (about 18 ounces total weight)
1 cup apple juice
1 teaspoon lemon juice
Pinch of grated lemon peel
Pinch of pumpkin-pie spice
2/3 cup golden raisins
1/4 cup chopped walnuts
3 large eggs plus 4 egg whites
3 tablespoons skim milk
1 teaspoon vanilla extract
1/4 teaspoon ground cinnamon
1 tablespoon plus 2 teaspoons vegetable oil
12 slices whole-wheat bread

Cook the apples, apple juice, lemon juice, peel and pumpkin-pie spice in a medium-size saucepan over medium heat for 10 minutes; process in a food processor or blender until puréed but still chunky. Stir in the raisins and walnuts, return the purée to the pan and cover to keep warm. In a large, shallow bowl whisk together the eggs, egg whites and milk. Add the vanilla and cinnamon. Heat 2 teaspoons of oil in a large nonstick skillet over medium-high heat. Dip 4 slices of bread into the egg mixture, place them in the skillet and cook for 3 minutes. Turn the toast and cook for another 3 minutes, or until well browned. Dip and cook the remaining bread in the same fashion, adding oil as necessary. Cut each piece of French toast into 4 strips, divide them among 6 plates and top each serving with apple purée.   Makes 6 servings

French Toast Fingers with Apple Purée

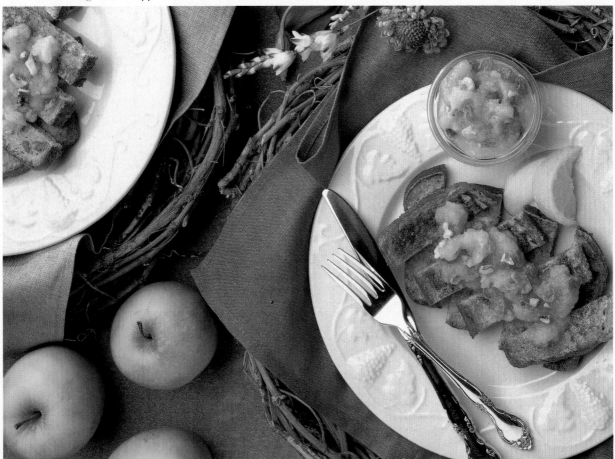

OATMEAL-BULGUR CEREAL WITH TANGERINES

Bulgur and oats are good sources of iron, a mineral that is often lacking in low-calorie diets. Tangerines contribute vitamin C, which aids in the absorption of iron, and they also provide your daily vitamin A requirement.

CALORIES per serving	363
74% Carbohydrate	69 g
15% Protein	14 g
11% Fat	4 g
CALCIUM	195 mg
IRON	3 mg
SODIUM	98 mg

3/4 cup coarse-cut bulgur
2 cups rolled oats
Pinch of salt
1/4 teaspoon ground cinnamon

2 cups lowfat milk (1%)
4 tangerines, peeled and sectioned
1 teaspoon grated lime peel

Place the bulgur in a medium-size bowl, add 1 cup of hot water and set aside for about 20 minutes, or until the bulgur is slightly softened.

Place the oats in a medium-size saucepan and add the salt, bulgur and 1 quart of water. Bring to a boil over medium heat and cook for 5 minutes, then reduce the heat to low and simmer for another 3 minutes, or until the cereal is thickened. Stir in the cinnamon, then spoon the cereal into 4 bowls and pour 1/2 cup of milk over each serving. Top the cereal with tangerine sections, sprinkle with lime peel and serve.   Makes 4 servings

WHOLE-GRAIN SODA BREAD

The whole grains in this bread provide insoluble fiber, which may help prevent some types of cancer, and the oats, nuts and raisins contain a type of fiber that has been shown to lower elevated blood cholesterol levels. High-fiber breads keep you feeling full longer than refined flour products do.

CALORIES per serving	336
70% Carbohydrate	62 g
10% Protein	9 g
20% Fat	8 g
CALCIUM	164 mg
IRON	3 mg
SODIUM	434 mg

1/4 cup wheat berries
3/4 cup dark raisins
Vegetable cooking spray
1 cup whole-wheat flour
1/2 cup all-purpose flour
1/2 cup rolled oats
1/4 cup chopped walnuts
1/4 cup dark brown sugar

2 teaspoons caraway seeds
2 teaspoons baking powder
1 teaspoon baking soda
1/4 teaspoon salt
1 cup plus 2 teaspoons buttermilk
1 large egg
1 tablespoon oil
1/4 cup honey

Place the wheat berries in a small bowl, add 1/2 cup of boiling water and set aside to soak for 1 hour, or until soft. Place the raisins in another small bowl, add hot water to cover and set aside to soak.

Preheat the oven to 375° F. Lightly spray a 9-inch round baking pan with cooking spray; set aside. Drain the wheat berries and raisins. In a large bowl stir together the whole-wheat flour, all-purpose flour, oats, walnuts, sugar, caraway seeds, baking powder, baking soda and salt; make a well in the center. Pour in 1 cup of buttermilk, the egg and oil and stir to blend. Add the drained wheat berries and raisins and stir just until the mixture forms a soft dough; do not overmix. Spoon the dough into the prepared pan, mounding it slightly in the center, and brush it with the remaining 2 teaspoons of buttermilk. Bake the bread in the center of the oven for 35 to 40 minutes, or until the loaf is golden brown and sounds hollow when removed from the pan and tapped on the bottom. Transfer the loaf to a wire rack to cool for 10 minutes, then cut it into 12 wedges and serve with honey.   Makes 6 servings

TORTILLAS RANCHERAS

Vegetables and beans make this Tex-Mex dish a fiber-rich brunch. If you use canned beans, rinse and drain them to reduce the sodium content.

CALORIES per serving	316
59% Carbohydrate	48 g
17% Protein	14 g
24% Fat	9 g
CALCIUM	125 mg
IRON	6 mg
SODIUM	20 mg

1 1/2 cups diced plum tomatoes
1 cup diced yellow bell pepper
1 cup diced red bell pepper
1/2 cup finely chopped scallions
1/4 cup chopped fresh coriander
1/4 cup freshly squeezed lime juice
Pinch of grated lime peel
1/2 teaspoon chili powder
1/2 teaspoon ground cumin
Pinch of red pepper flakes, or to taste
1 1/2 cups cooked black beans (3/4 cup dried)
2 teaspoons vegetable oil
Four 7-inch flour tortillas
3 cups shredded Romaine lettuce
1/3 cup unsalted roasted peanuts

In a medium-size bowl stir together the tomatoes, bell peppers, scallions, coriander, lime juice, lime peel, chili powder, cumin and pepper flakes. Add the black beans and stir to combine; set aside.

Heat 1/2 teaspoon of oil in a medium-size nonstick skillet over medium-high heat. Place a tortilla in the skillet and cook for about 1 minute on each side, or until it is warmed and softened. Repeat with the remaining tortillas and place them on 4 plates. Top each tortilla with shredded lettuce, spoon the tomato mixture on top and sprinkle with peanuts.   Makes 4 servings

COUSCOUS-CURRANT CEREAL

For this unusual hot breakfast cereal, couscous, a tiny, grain-like pasta made from semolina flour, is cooked in apple juice.

CALORIES per serving	310
86% Carbohydrate	59 g
13% Protein	9 g
1% Fat	3 g
CALCIUM	101 mg
IRON	1 mg
SODIUM	37 mg

2 cups apple juice
Pinch of ground cinnamon
1 cup instant couscous
1/2 cup dried currants
1 cup skim milk
4 strawberries, washed and hulled

Place the apple juice and cinnamon in a small saucepan and bring to a boil over high heat. Remove the pan from the heat, add the couscous and currants and cover the pan; set aside for 5 minutes. Meanwhile, warm the milk in another small saucepan over medium-low heat.

Fluff the couscous with a fork and divide it among 4 bowls. Top each serving with a strawberry and serve with the warm milk.   Makes 4 servings

STRAWBERRY-ORANGE MILK SHAKE ▼

No sugar is added to this breakfast drink. It gets its sweetness — and its abundance of vitamin C and the mineral potassium — from fresh fruit.

CALORIES per serving	124
81% Carbohydrate	26 g
11% Protein	4 g
8% Fat	1 g
CALCIUM	97 mg
IRON	1 mg
SODIUM	67 mg

1 cup sliced strawberries
1 cup orange juice
1/2 small banana
1/2 cup buttermilk

Combine all the ingredients in a blender and process until smoothly blended. Pour the mixture into 2 tall glasses and serve.   Makes 2 servings

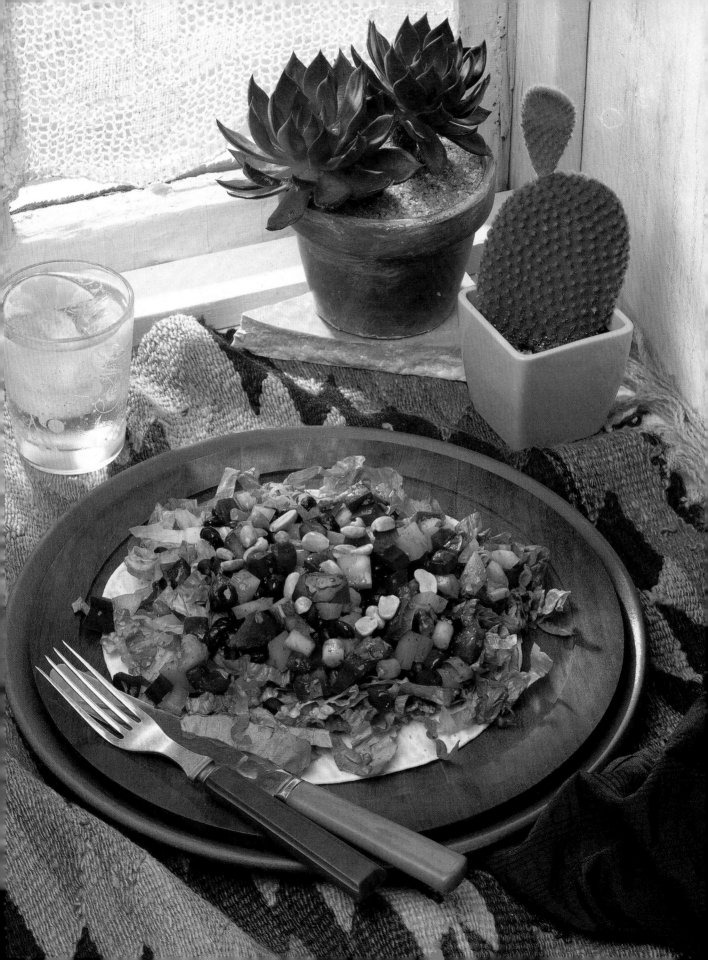

CORNMEAL-CHEESE ENGLISH MUFFINS

CALORIES per serving	367
69% Carbohydrate	64 g
14% Protein	13 g
17% Fat	5 g
CALCIUM	126 mg
IRON	3 mg
SODIUM	444 mg

The ricotta topping served with these muffins is a good lowfat source of calcium. Butter, on the other hand, derives 100 percent of its calories from fat and provides no significant nutrients except vitamin A.

1 cup frozen corn kernels
1 1/4 cups unbleached all-purpose flour, approximately
1 cup cornmeal, approximately
1 cup whole-wheat flour
3/4 teaspoon salt
3/4 teaspoon pepper
1/4 cup blue cheese, crumbled
1 large egg white
2 teaspoons vegetable oil
1 package dry yeast
1 1/2 tablespoons honey
1/2 cup part skim-milk ricotta cheese
2 tablespoons finely chopped scallions

Place the corn in a food processor and process for about 10 seconds, or until chopped. Remove about half of the corn and set aside. Add 1 1/4 cups of all-purpose flour, 1 cup of cornmeal, the whole-wheat flour, salt, pepper, blue cheese, egg white and oil to the food processor and cover it; set aside. Place the yeast in a small cup, add 1/4 cup warm water (105-115° F) and 1/2 tablespoon of honey and set aside for about 5 minutes, or until foamy.

Stir the yeast mixture. Start the food processor, pour in the yeast mixture through the feed tube and process for about 40 seconds. Add the reserved chopped corn kernels and process for another 5 seconds; the dough should form a ball. Place the dough in a medium-size bowl, cover it with a kitchen towel and set aside in a warm place to rise for 1 hour, or until the dough is doubled in bulk.

Sprinkle a baking sheet with 2 teaspoons of cornmeal. Punch down the dough and on a lightly floured board roll it out to a 3/8-inch thickness. Using a 3 1/2-inch biscuit cutter, cut out 6 rounds. Transfer the muffins to the baking sheet, cover with a towel and set aside in a warm place to rise for 25 minutes, or until the muffins are about 1 1/2 times their original size.

Heat a medium-size nonstick skillet over medium heat. Using a metal spatula place 3 muffins in the skillet and cook for about 6 minutes, or until the bottoms of the muffins are golden brown. Turn the muffins and cook for another 6 minutes. Transfer the cooked muffins to a wire rack to cool and cook the remaining muffins in the same fashion.

Just before serving, stir together the ricotta and scallions in a small bowl. Split and toast the muffins, then spread each half with 2 teaspoons of the ricotta spread and serve. Makes 6 servings

Note: The muffins can be made ahead and frozen, but the spread should be made shortly before serving, or the flavor of the scallions may become unpleasantly strong.

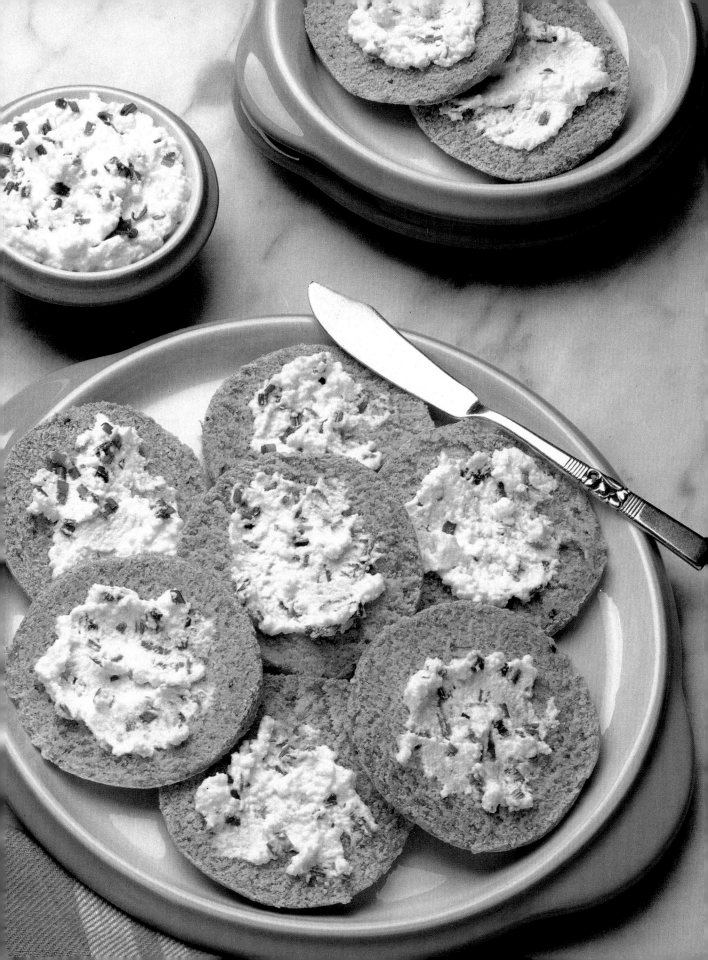

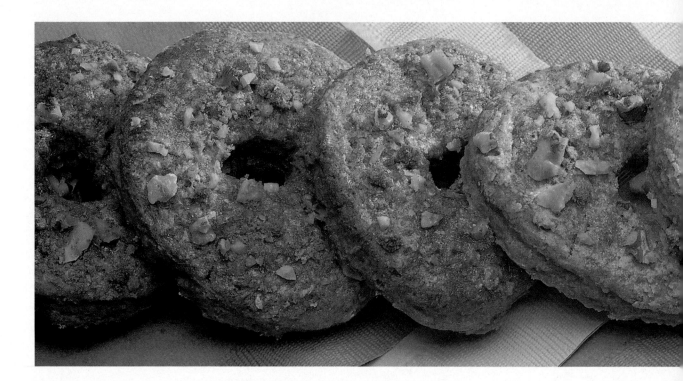

BAKED SWEET POTATO DOUGHNUTS

These doughnuts are filling because of their healthfully high fiber content. And because they are baked rather than deep fried, they are more quickly digested than regular doughnuts.

CALORIES per doughnut	275
66% Carbohydrate	46 g
9% Protein	7 g
25% Fat	8 g
CALCIUM	109 mg
IRON	2 mg
SODIUM	329 mg

1 sweet potato (about 6 ounces)
1 cup unbleached all-purpose
   flour, approximately
3/4 cup whole-wheat flour
2 teaspoons baking powder
1 teaspoon ground cinnamon
1/2 teaspoon baking soda
1/4 teaspoon ground nutmeg

1/4 teaspoon salt
1 large egg plus 1 large egg white
2 tablespoons vegetable oil
5 tablespoons light brown sugar
2 tablespoons frozen apple juice
   concentrate, thawed
Vegetable cooking spray
2 tablespoons chopped walnuts

Place the sweet potato in a small saucepan with cold water to cover and bring to a boil over medium-high heat. Cook the potato for about 35 minutes, or until fork-tender; drain. When the potato is cool enough to handle, peel it, place it in a large bowl and mash it; set aside.

Preheat the oven to 425° F. In a small bowl stir together 1 cup of the all-purpose flour, the whole-wheat flour, baking powder, cinnamon, baking soda, nutmeg and salt; set aside. In another small bowl beat the egg white with a fork; add 1 tablespoon of the beaten white to the mashed potato. Reserve the remainder of the egg white. Add the whole egg, oil, 4 tablespoons of brown sugar and the apple juice concentrate to the mashed potato and mix until well blended. Add the dry ingredients and stir to form a dough.

Spray a baking sheet with cooking spray; set aside. Turn the dough out onto a lightly floured board, knead it a few times and roll it out to a 3/8-inch

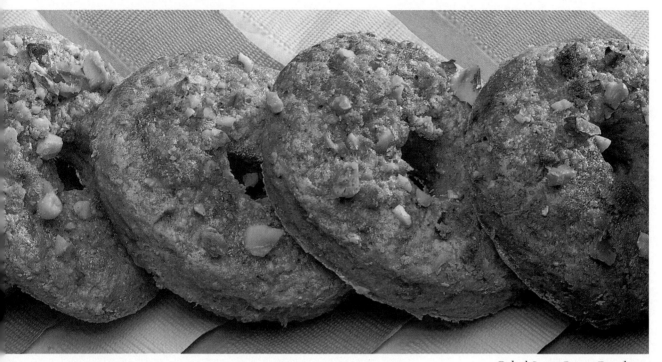

Baked Sweet Potato Doughnuts

thickness. Using a 3-inch doughnut cutter, cut out 6 doughnuts. Combine the walnuts and remaining sugar on a small plate. (For less sweet doughnuts, omit the sugar from the topping.) Brush the tops of the doughnuts and the cut-out centers with the remaining egg white, dip them in the walnut topping and place them on the baking sheet. Bake the doughnuts for 13 to 15 minutes, or until the tops are golden and the bottoms are lightly browned. Transfer the doughnuts to a rack to cool briefly and serve warm.   Makes 6 servings

FRUIT WITH LEMON YOGURT SAUCE

A variety of fresh fruits can help to keep low-calorie meals interesting while providing important nutrients. Each generous serving of this fruit salad provides one fourth the calcium, one third the phosphorus and all the vitamins A and C you need daily; in addition it supplies a good amount of potassium.

CALORIES per serving	356
60% Carbohydrate	58 g
11% Protein	11 g
29% Fat	12 g
CALCIUM	272 mg
IRON	2 mg
SODIUM	100 mg

1 cup plain lowfat yogurt
1 tablespoon granulated sugar
2 teaspoons lemon juice
1 1/2 teaspoons grated lemon peel
1 cup diced cantaloupe
1 cup diced honeydew

1 cup diced fresh pineapple
1 cup sliced fresh strawberries
1/2 cup fresh raspberries
1/2 cup seedless red grapes
1/2 cup diced papaya
1/4 cup chopped walnuts

For the sauce, in a small bowl stir together the yogurt, sugar, lemon juice and lemon peel; set aside. Place all the fruit in a large bowl and toss gently to combine. Divide the fruit mixture between 2 bowls, top each serving with half the sauce and sprinkle with walnuts.   Makes 2 servings

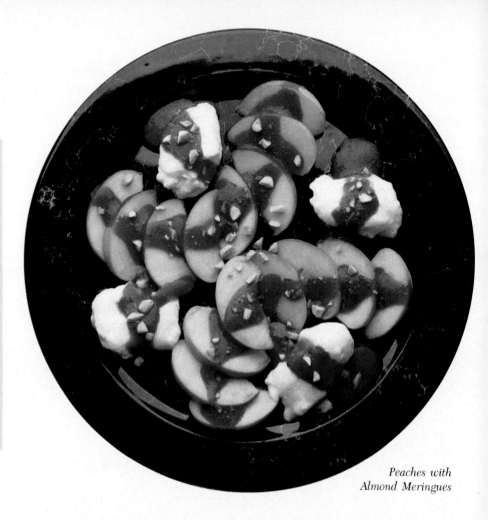

*Peaches with
Almond Meringues*

PEACHES WITH ALMOND MERINGUES ▼

For low-calorie cooking, try to use more egg whites than yolks: A large egg white has 3 grams of protein, no fat and no cholesterol, while the yolk has nearly 6 grams of fat and about 275 milligrams of cholesterol.

CALORIES per serving	201
70% Carbohydrate	38 g
12% Protein	6 g
18% Fat	4 g
CALCIUM	35 mg
IRON	1 mg
SODIUM	51 mg

4 black plums, halved and pitted
Pinch of cinnamon
4 peaches, halved and pitted

4 egg whites, at room temperature
1/4 cup sugar
12 whole toasted almonds, chopped

For the sauce, coarsely chop the plums. Process them with the cinnamon in a food processor or blender for 1 minute, or until smooth. Strain the sauce; set aside. Cut the peaches into 1/2-inch-thick slices; set aside.

For the meringues, fill a large skillet three-quarters full of water and bring it to a simmer over medium heat. Meanwhile, in a large bowl, using an electric mixer, beat the egg whites until firm but not dry. Whisk in the sugar 1 tablespoon at a time, then whisk the egg whites for another 30 seconds, or until glossy. Make the meringues in 2 batches: Carefully place 8 separate heaping tablespoons of meringue in the simmering water and poach them for about 10 seconds, then flip them over and poach them for another 5 seconds, or just until firm. Using a slotted spoon, transfer the meringues to a plate. Make another 8 meringues in the same fashion. Arrange the peach slices and the meringues on 4 plates, spoon some plum sauce over each serving and sprinkle with almonds. Makes 4 servings

HOMINY HASH

Canned corned-beef hash derives about 60 percent of its calories from fat, but this hash, based on hominy (hulled corn) and vegetables flavored with a small amount of bacon, has a much healthier carbohydrate-fat balance. Canned hominy should be rinsed to reduce its sodium content.

CALORIES per serving	305
63% Carbohydrate	50 g
10% Protein	8 g
27% Fat	10 g
CALCIUM	41 mg
IRON	4 mg
SODIUM	912 mg

2 medium-size potatoes, peeled and coarsely diced

2 tablespoons olive oil

2 medium-size onions, peeled and coarsely diced

2 medium-size green bell peppers, seeded and coarsely diced

2 teaspoons cumin seed

4 cups canned yellow hominy, rinsed and drained

1/2 teaspoon black pepper

Hot pepper sauce to taste

2 slices Canadian bacon, diced

2 medium-size tomatoes, coarsely diced

4 scallions, thinly sliced

Bring a medium-size saucepan of water to a boil over medium-high heat, add the potatoes and cook for 10 minutes, or until soft. Drain the potatoes and dry the pan. In a large bowl mash the potatoes lightly with a fork; they should not be completely smooth. Heat 2 teaspoons of oil in the saucepan over medium-high heat. Add the onions and bell peppers and cook, stirring, for 3 minutes, or until the vegetables begin to wilt. Add 2 tablespoons of water, cover, reduce the heat to low and cook for 10 minutes, or until the vegetables are soft. Meanwhile, toast the cumin seeds in a small dry skillet over high heat, shaking the skillet, for 1 minute, or until the seeds are fragrant and brown. Chop the seeds and add to the potatoes along with the cooked vegetables, hominy, black pepper, hot pepper sauce and bacon; mix well.

Preheat the oven to 200° F. Divide the hash into 4 equal portions. Heat 1 teaspoon of oil in a medium-size nonstick skillet over high heat. Add 1 portion of hash and press it with a spatula to form a flat patty. Cook for 2 minutes, or until the patty is browned on the bottom, then turn it and cook for another 2 to 3 minutes, or until browned. Transfer the patty to an ovenproof plate and keep it warm in the oven. Repeat with the remaining hash. Divide the patties among 4 plates and top them with tomatoes and scallions.   Makes 4 servings

QUICK OATS WITH MIXED FRUIT

Quick-cooking oats have the same amount of cholesterol-lowering oat bran as old-fashioned oatmeal — in fact, the two are nutritionally identical.

CALORIES per serving	302
84% Carbohydrate	67 g
10% Protein	8 g
6% Fat	2 g
CALCIUM	33 mg
IRON	2 mg
SODIUM	118 mg

3/4 cup apple juice

2/3 cup quick-cooking oats

Pinch of salt

Pinch of ground cinnamon

1/3 cup mixed dried fruit, finely chopped

2 tablespoons honey

2/3 cup skim milk

In a small saucepan stir together the apple juice, oats, salt, cinnamon and 3/4 cup of water and bring to a boil over medium-high heat. Reduce the heat to low, cover the pan and simmer for 1 minute, or until the liquid is absorbed; remove the pan from the heat. Stir in the fruit and honey, cover the pan and let stand for 2 minutes, or until the fruit is softened. Divide the oatmeal between 2 bowls and pour some milk over each serving.   Makes 2 servings

FRUIT AND RICE FRITTERS ▼

CALORIES per fritter	221
65% Carbohydrate	38 g
9% Protein	5 g
26% Fat	7 g
CALCIUM	28 mg
IRON	2 mg
SODIUM	121 mg

Fritters are, by definition, fried. But these fritters are cooked in just a fraction of the oil needed for deep frying. The dried fruit and brown rice supply fiber and important minerals, notably iron and potassium.

5 dried pear halves

5 dried peach halves

5 dried apricots

4 tablespoons whole-wheat flour

1 1/2 cups cooked brown rice
   (1/2 cup raw)

1 large egg, separated, plus 2 large
   egg whites

1 tablespoon toasted sesame seeds

1/4 teaspoon salt

1/4 teaspoon pumpkin-pie spice

2 tablespoons vegetable oil

Finely chop the dried fruit, place it in a medium-size bowl with the flour and toss to coat the fruit. Add the rice, egg yolk, sesame seeds, salt and pumpkin-pie spice and mix well; set aside. In a large bowl, using an electric mixer, beat the egg whites until stiff. Gently fold them into the rice mixture. Heat the oil in a large nonstick skillet over medium heat. Using 1/2 cup of batter for each, make 3 fritters, flattening them with a spatula to a 1/2-inch thickness. Cook for 2 to 3 minutes, then turn and cook for another 2 to 3 minutes, or until the fritters are golden on both sides. Make 3 more fritters in the same fashion and serve immediately. Makes 6 servings

BREAKFAST INDIAN PUDDINGS

CALORIES per serving	329
70% Carbohydrate	58 g
14% Protein	11 g
16% Fat	6 g
CALCIUM	380 mg
IRON	6 mg
SODIUM	172 mg

Dark molasses, the traditional sweetener for this New England dish, is a source of calcium; the combination of molasses, milk and yogurt provides about one third of the daily requirement.

2/3 cup yellow cornmeal

1/4 cup dark molasses

2 large eggs

1 1/2 teapoons ground cinnamon

1 teaspoon ground ginger

1/2 teaspoon ground nutmeg

Pinch of salt

2 cups lowfat milk (2%)

1 cup apricot nectar

1 teaspoon vanilla extract

8 dried apricots

1/2 cup plain lowfat yogurt

Preheat the oven to 325° F. In a large bowl whisk together the cornmeal, molasses, eggs, 1 1/4 teaspoons of cinnamon, the ginger, nutmeg and salt; set aside. Heat the milk, apricot nectar and vanilla in a medium-size saucepan over medium-high heat until hot. Whisk 1 cup of the hot liquid into the corn-meal mixture, then whisk in the remaining liquid. Return the mixture to the saucepan and cook, whisking constantly, for 2 minutes, or until it thickens and starts to bubble. Divide the mixture among four 1-cup ramekins and bake for about 40 minutes, or until firm and browned on top.

Let the puddings cool at room temperature for about 30 minutes. (If making them the night before, cover and refrigerate them when cool; reheat them in a 350° F oven for 20 minutes.) A few minutes before serving, place the apricots in a small bowl and add boiling water to cover; let stand for 1 minute. Drain the apricots and cut them into strips. Top each pudding with 2 tablespoons of yogurt and some apricot strips and sprinkle with the remaining cinnamon.

Makes 4 servings

RASPBERRY FROZEN YOGURT FLOAT ▼

This soda fountain-style treat is rich in fiber and potassium. The frozen yogurt can also be served as a nutritious snack or dessert.

4 medium-size pears

2 cups fresh or frozen raspberries

3 cups plain lowfat yogurt

1 tablespoon pure maple syrup

1 egg white

1 quart salt-free seltzer

CALORIES per serving	250
71% Carbohydrate	47 g
17% Protein	11 g
12% Fat	4 g
CALCIUM	349 mg
IRON	1 mg
SODIUM	132 mg

Peel, core and dice the pears. Purée the raspberries in a food processor or blender; strain the purée into a small bowl and set aside. Purée the pears, then add the raspberry purée, yogurt, maple syrup and egg white, and process until thoroughly combined. Transfer the mixture to a shallow metal pan, cover with plastic wrap and place in the freezer overnight.

Let the frozen yogurt thaw at room temperature for 30 minutes, or until slightly softened. Scoop equal portions of the frozen yogurt into 4 tall glasses, add 8 ounces of seltzer to each and serve. Makes 4 servings

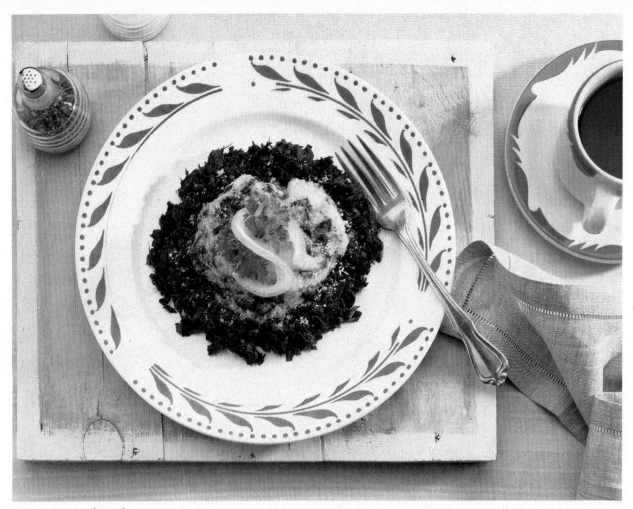

Cheese Grits with Garlic Greens

CHEESE GRITS WITH GARLIC GREENS

Dark leafy greens like beet tops are not only excellent sources of vitamin A and potassium, but are among the best nondairy sources of calcium as well.

2 tablespoons olive oil
8 garlic cloves, minced
4 cups cooked beet greens,
    chopped, or frozen beet greens,
    thawed, drained and chopped

1/2 cup chopped fresh parsley
2 1/2 cups instant grits
1/4 cup plus 2 tablespoons grated
    Parmesan
1 teaspoon pepper

Heat the oil in a medium-size saucepan over low heat, add the garlic and sauté for 2 minutes, or until fragrant. Add the beet greens, parsley and 3 tablespoons of water, cover and cook for 5 minutes, or until the greens are heated through. Meanwhile, in another medium-size saucepan bring 5 cups of water to a boil over high heat. Remove the pan from the heat, add the grits, 1/4 cup of Parmesan and the pepper, and stir until thick and well blended. Stir in half the greens. Divide the remaining greens among 6 plates and spoon the grits mixture on top. Sprinkle with the remaining Parmesan and serve.

Makes 6 servings

CALORIES per serving	342
69% Carbohydrate	59 g
13% Protein	11 g
18% Fat	7 g
CALCIUM	195 mg
IRON	5 mg
SODIUM	328 mg

PINEAPPLE-OATMEAL MUFFINS ▼

Wrap the muffins individually and freeze them, then thaw one at a time as a take-along breakfast. If you usually stop en route to work for a croissant or pastry, you will save minutes as well as calories.

Vegetable cooking spray (optional)
2 cups unbleached
   all-purpose flour
2 teaspoons baking powder
2 1/4 teaspoons ground ginger
2 1/4 teaspoons ground cinnamon
3 large eggs, lightly beaten

6 slices unsweetened dried
   pineapple, finely chopped
3/4 cup pineapple juice
1/4 cup honey
1 tablespoon plus 1 teaspoon
   vegetable oil
1 1/2 teaspoons vanilla extract
1 cup rolled oats

Preheat the oven to 400° F. Lightly spray 12 muffin tin cups with cooking spray or line them with paper liners; set aside. Sift the flour, baking powder, ginger and cinnamon into a medium-size bowl; set aside. In a large bowl stir together the eggs, pineapple, pineapple juice, honey, oil and vanilla. Stir in the sifted dry ingredients and the oats and stir just until combined: Do not overmix. Divide the batter among the muffin tin cups and bake for 20 minutes, or until a toothpick inserted in the center of a muffin comes out clean. Transfer the muffins to a rack to cool. If you are freezing the muffins, wrap them individually in plastic wrap when completely cooled.   Makes 12 muffins

CALORIES per muffin	187
72% Carbohydrate	34 g
11% Protein	5 g
17% Fat	4 g
CALCIUM	60 mg
IRON	2 mg
SODIUM	90 mg

JOHNNYCAKES WITH BLUEBERRY SAUCE

Johnnycakes are light, crisp cornmeal pancakes made without eggs or butter. The cooked berries are naturally sweet without added sugar, making them a healthier topping than syrups that are virtually pure sugar.

1 1/2 cups fresh blueberries,
   washed, or frozen unsweetened
   blueberries, thawed
2 tablespoons orange juice
1/2 teaspoon grated orange peel

1 cup cornmeal
Pinch of salt
1/4 cup skim milk
1 tablespoon vegetable oil

For the sauce, combine the blueberries, orange juice and orange peel in a medium-size nonreactive saucepan and cook over medium heat, stirring and mashing the berries with a wooden spoon, for 7 to 10 minutes, or until the sauce is thick and syrupy. Remove the pan from the heat and cover it to keep the sauce warm; set aside.

   Bring a small saucepan of water to a boil. In a large bowl stir together the cornmeal and salt. Add 1 1/4 cups of boiling water and mix well, then stir in the milk. Heat the oil in a heavy nonstick skillet over medium heat. Using a scant 1/4 cup of batter for each, make 4 pancakes. Cook the pancakes for 3 minutes, or until they are golden on the bottom, then turn them and cook for another 3 to 5 minutes, or until golden and crisp. Transfer the pancakes to a plate. Using the remaining batter make another 4 pancakes in the same fashion and place them on a second plate. Pour the blueberry sauce over the johnnycakes and serve.   Makes 2 servings

CALORIES per serving	391
74% Carbohydrate	73 g
7% Protein	7 g
19% Fat	8 g
CALCIUM	51 mg
IRON	2 mg
SODIUM	89 mg

Artificial sweeteners may not help you lose weight; in fact, they may hinder your efforts at weight control. The sweeteners do not satisfy hunger, and in some people they actually stimulate feelings of hunger. A study has shown that long-time users of artificial sweeteners are more likely to gain weight in the course of a year than people who do not use the sweeteners, and they are more likely to gain more weight (more than 16 percent of body weight) than nonusers.

GINGERBREAD-BROWN RICE PANCAKES ▼

When you include lowfat dairy products such as buttermilk and part skim-milk ricotta in your breakfast dishes, you keep your calorie, fat and cholesterol intakes low and get plenty of calcium as well.

1/2 cup brown rice	3/4 teaspoon ground cinnamon
2 tablespoons lemon juice	1/2 teaspoon ground cloves
2 tablespoons honey	3/4 cup buttermilk
2 teaspoons cornstarch	3 tablespoons molasses
1 cup unbleached all-purpose flour	2 egg whites
1/4 cup chopped walnuts	1 tablespoon grated fresh ginger
1 teaspoon baking powder	1/4 cup part skim-milk ricotta
1/2 teaspoon baking soda	cheese

Bring 1 1/4 cups of water to a boil in a small saucepan over medium heat. Add the rice, cover the pan, reduce the heat to low and cook for 30 minutes, or until the rice is just tender and the water is absorbed. Remove the pan from the heat and let cool until the rice is just warm. (You can also cook the rice in advance or use 1 1/2 cups leftover rice.)

Meanwhile, for the sauce, in a small saucepan stir together the lemon juice, honey, cornstarch and 2 tablespoons of water. Bring the sauce to a boil over medium heat, stirring constantly, and boil for 30 seconds, or until the sauce thickens. Remove the pan from the heat and set aside to cool.

Stir together the flour, walnuts, baking powder, baking soda, cinnamon and cloves in a large bowl and make a well in the center. Pour in the buttermilk, molasses, egg whites and ginger and stir until combined. Stir the rice to break it up, then add it to the batter and stir just until combined.

Preheat the oven to 200° F. Heat a medium-size nonstick skillet over medium-low heat. Using 2 tablespoons of batter for each, make 3 pancakes. Cook for 3 minutes, or until bubbles form on the tops of the pancakes, then turn them and cook for another 3 minutes, or until golden. Transfer the pancakes to a heatproof platter, cover with foil and place in the oven to keep warm. Make another 5 batches of pancakes in the same fashion.

To serve, fold the ricotta into the sauce. Divide the pancakes among 6 plates and top each serving with a heaping tablespoon of sauce.

Makes 6 servings

CALORIES per serving	245
71% Carbohydrate	44 g
12% Protein	7 g
17% Fat	5 g
CALCIUM	189 mg
IRON	3 mg
SODIUM	215 mg

CARROT-BUTTERMILK SHAKE

This drink combines carrots and apricots, both rich in vitamin A, with lowfat buttermilk, which adds high-quality protein. The apple, carrots and nuts provide fiber and give this filling meal in a glass a rich, thick texture.

1 small McIntosh apple (5 ounces)	1/2 teaspoon grated fresh ginger
1 cup sliced, cooked carrots	1 1/2 cups buttermilk
2 tablespoons chopped walnuts	1 cup apricot nectar
2 tablespoons dark brown sugar	2 ice cubes

Peel and core the apple and cut it into large chunks. Place the apple and all the remaining ingredients in a food processor or blender and process until smooth. Pour the shake into 2 tall glasses and serve.   *Makes 2 servings*

CALORIES per serving	313
71% Carbohydrate	59 g
11% Protein	9 g
18% Fat	7 g
CALCIUM	267 mg
IRON	2 mg
SODIUM	253 mg

*Brown Rice Cereal
with Fruit and Almonds*

BROWN RICE CEREAL WITH FRUIT AND ALMONDS

*Brown rice, apricots, almonds and an unpeeled apple provide a fiber-rich
breakfast with none of the refined sweeteners (sugar, dextrose or corn
syrup) usually added to packaged breakfast cereals.*

CALORIES per serving	363
70% Carbohydrate	64 g
11% Protein	10 g
19% Fat	8 g
CALCIUM	159 mg
IRON	2 mg
SODIUM	71 mg

2 cups brown rice

1/4 teaspoon ground allspice

Pinch of salt

1/2 cup dried apricots, cut into
   thin strips

1/2 cup slivered toasted almonds

1 Delicious apple, cored
   and chopped

2 cups lowfat milk (2%)

Place the rice, allspice, salt and 1 quart of water in a medium-size saucepan
and bring to a boil over medium heat. Cover the pan, reduce the heat to low
and cook for 40 minutes, or until the rice is tender and the water is absorbed.
Add the apricots and cook for another 5 minutes. Divide the cereal among 4
bowls, sprinkle with almonds and chopped apple, and pour 1/2 cup of milk over
each serving.   Makes 6 servings

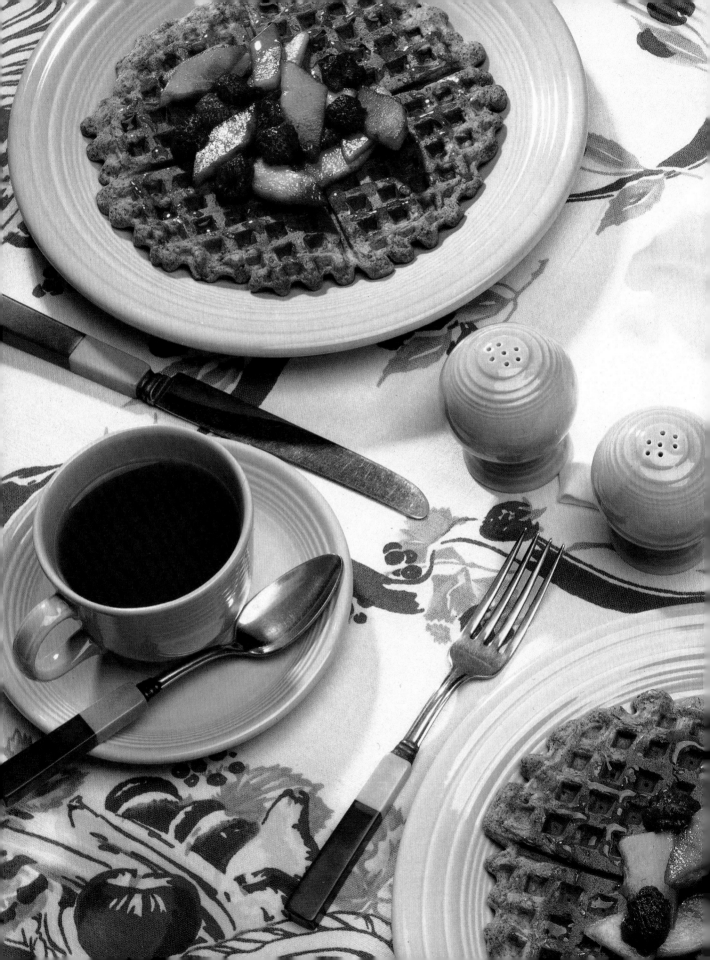

BUCKWHEAT-WILD RICE WAFFLES

Egg whites can be substituted for whole eggs in many waffle and pancake recipes, thereby cutting fat and cholesterol. These waffles have an especially hearty flavor thanks to the combination of buckwheat and wild rice.

CALORIES per serving	**300**
70% Carbohydrate	53 g
11% Protein	9 g
19% Fat	7 g
CALCIUM	174 mg
IRON	2 mg
SODIUM	293 mg

1 cup unbleached all-purpose flour

3/4 cup light buckwheat flour

2 teaspoons baking powder

1/4 teaspoon salt

3 tablespoons honey

2 tablespoons vegetable oil

1 1/2 cups lowfat milk (2%)

Vegetable cooking spray

3 large egg whites

3/4 cup cold cooked wild rice
   (about 3 tablespoons raw)

1 cup thinly sliced cantaloupe

1 cup fresh raspberries or frozen
   unsweetened raspberries, thawed

3 tablespoons pure maple syrup

For the waffles, in a large bowl stir together the flours, baking powder and salt and make a well in the center. Pour in the honey and oil and and mix until blended. Add the milk and stir until the batter is until fairly smooth; set aside.

Preheat the oven to 200° F. Spray a nonstick waffle iron with cooking spray and preheat it. In a large bowl, using an electric mixer, beat the egg whites until soft peaks form. Gently fold the egg whites into the batter, then fold in the wild rice. Pour 1 cup of batter into the waffle iron and cook for 2 to 3 minutes, or according to the manufacturer's instructions, until the waffle is golden. Transfer the waffle to an ovenproof platter and place it in the oven to keep warm. Using the remaining batter, make 5 more waffles in the same fashion. (Do not respray the hot waffle iron with cooking spray.)

Divide the waffles among 6 plates, top them with melon and berries, and drizzle 1 1/2 teaspoons of maple syrup over each waffle.   Makes 6 servings

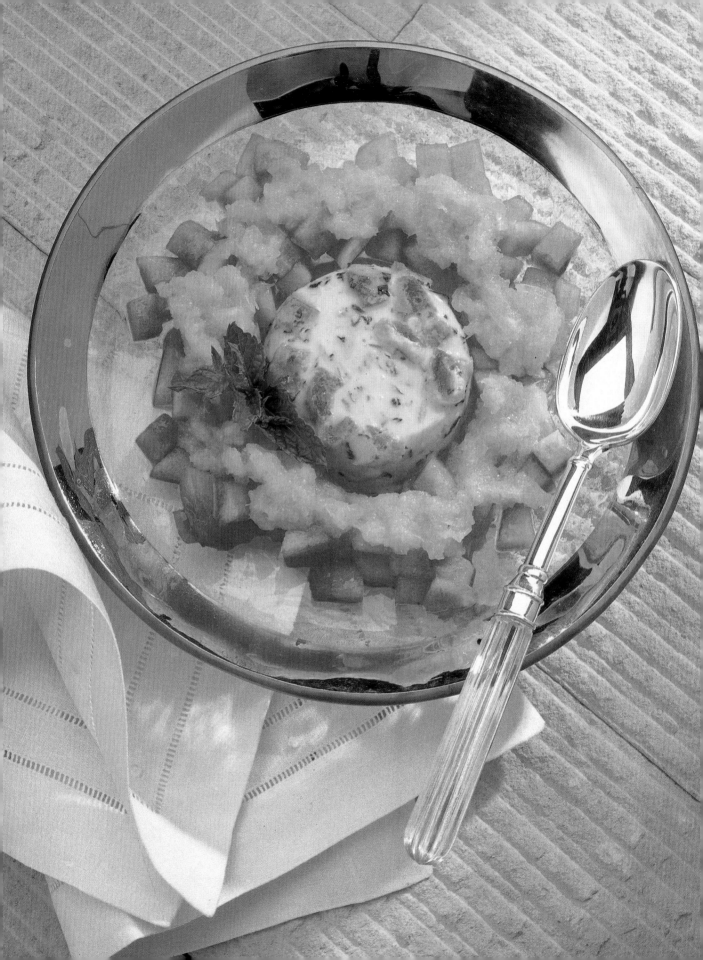

RICOTTA MOUSSE WITH CHUNKY PINEAPPLE SAUCE

A mousse may seem like an unusual breakfast, but this combination of fruit and lowfat dairy products makes a nice change of pace. The cantaloupe provides a full day's supply of vitamins A and C.

CALORIES per serving	323
65% Carbohydrate	55 g
15% Protein	13 g
20% Fat	8 g
CALCIUM	257 mg
IRON	2 mg
SODIUM	117 mg

1 large egg yolk
1/2 cup lowfat milk (2%)
1/4 cup sugar
1 envelope unflavored gelatin
1 teaspoon grated orange peel
1 cup part skim-milk ricotta
   cheese
1/2 cup orange juice
1/4 teaspoon vanilla extract

1/2 cup chopped fresh mint leaves,
   plus 4 mint sprigs for garnish
1/4 cup chopped dried apricots
1 1/2 cups drained juice-packed
   pineapple chunks
6 tablespoons lemon juice
1 teaspoon grated lemon peel
One cantaloupe, peeled,
   seeded and chopped (4 cups)

Bring enough water to a simmer in the bottom pan of a double boiler so that the simmering water will not touch the top pan. For the mousse, place the egg yolk and milk in the top pan and cook, whisking constantly, over the simmering water for 10 minutes, or until the mixture begins to thicken slightly. Add the sugar, gelatin and orange peel, and cook, stirring constantly, for 8 minutes, or until the mixture is quite thick. Transfer to a medium-size bowl and set aside to cool for about 15 minutes.

Meanwhile, place the ricotta, orange juice and vanilla in a food processor or blender and process for 1 minute. Add the chopped mint and process for another 20 seconds. Fold the ricotta mixture into the gelatin mixture, then fold in the apricots until well blended. Spoon the mousse into four 4-ounce custard cups, cover and refrigerate for at least 1 hour, or overnight.

For the sauce combine the pineapple, lemon juice and lemon peel in a small saucepan and cook over medium heat for 5 minutes, then transfer the mixture to a food processor or blender and process for 10 seconds, or just until roughly chopped. Cover and refrigerate the sauce until ready to serve.

To unmold the mousses, dip each custard cup in a bowl of hot water for 10 to 15 seconds, then invert it on a plate. Surround each mousse with 1 cup of cantaloupe and spoon some of the pineapple sauce over the cantaloupe.

Makes 4 servings

R *ather than concentrating on those foods you must avoid, look for less familiar but nutritious foods to add variety to your diet. Many of the more exotic fruits — such as papayas, mangoes, kiwi fruits, pomegranates, Asian pears, star fruits, kumquats and passion fruits — are good low-calorie sources of vitamins A and C and potassium as well as fiber. These fruits are becoming more widely available in supermarkets.*

FRUIT GAZPACHO COOLER

Some soft drinks contain fruit juice and modest amounts of vitamin C: This tart refresher has nearly the full daily requirement of vitamin C and a good amount of vitamin A — and has no refined sugar or artificial sweetener.

1/4 cup washed, stemmed
   seedless grapes
1/2 cup low-sodium tomato juice

1/4 cup freshly squeezed
   orange juice
1 tablespoon sour cream

CALORIES per serving	108
66% Carbohydrate	19 g
7% Protein	2 g
27% Fat	3 g
CALCIUM	39 mg
IRON	1 mg
SODIUM	21 mg

Spread the grapes on a small plate and place them in the freezer for 2 hours, or until frozen solid. Place the tomato juice and orange juice in a blender and start the machine, then add the grapes and process until coarsely chopped. Pour the drink into a glass, top with sour cream and serve. Makes 1 serving

◁ *Ricotta Mousse with Chunky Pineapple Sauce*

Mid-Morning Snacks

OATMEAL BANANA BARS

CALORIES per bar	77
75% Carbohydrate	15 g
10% Protein	2 g
15% Fat	1 g
CALCIUM	11 mg
IRON	1 mg
SODIUM	7 mg

This snack cake is sweetened with banana, currants, unsweetened apple juice — and just one tablespoon of sugar. By comparison, commercial frozen banana cake contains more sugar, by weight, than any other ingredient, and derives 36 percent of its calories from fat.

Vegetable cooking spray
1 tablespoon whipped margarine
1 tablespoon brown sugar
1 cup rolled oats
1/4 teaspoon ground cinnamon

1/2 cup whole-wheat flour
1/2 cup apple juice
1/2 teaspoon vanilla extract
1 banana, mashed
1/4 cup dried currants

Preheat the oven to 350° F. Spray an 8-inch square baking pan with cooking spray. In a medium-size bowl beat together the margarine and sugar until creamy. Stir in the oats and cinnamon until combined, then add the flour and stir until combined. Mix the apple juice, vanilla and 1/2 cup of warm water in a small bowl, then add this mixture to the dry ingredients and stir well. Stir in the mashed banana and currants. Spread the dough in the prepared pan, smoothing the top with a rubber spatula, and bake for about 1 hour, or until the top is golden. Let the cake cool in the pan on a rack. To serve, cut the cake into quarters, then cut each quarter into 3 bars.   Makes 12 servings

Rye-Cheese Crackers

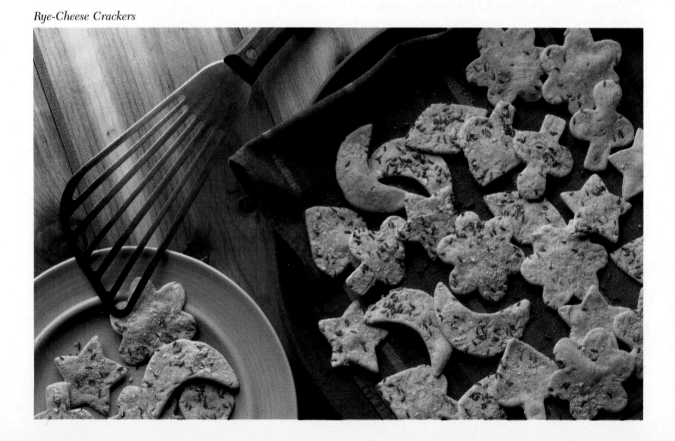

CRANBERRY POACHED PEARS WITH YOGURT

Low-calorie diets, especially those that include little meat, are often deficient in iron. Cranberry juice contains iron, and each serving of this dish supplies more than 45 milligrams of vitamin C, which helps the body use the iron.

1 cup unsweetened cranberry juice	1 cinnamon stick
1 teaspoon sugar	2 whole cloves
1 teaspoon grated lemon peel	1 large pear, peeled, halved and cored
1/2 teaspoon grated orange peel	1/2 cup plain lowfat yogurt
1/2 teaspoon vanilla extract	1 tablespoon toasted sesame seeds

CALORIES per serving	166
73% Carbohydrate	32 g
10% Protein	4 g
17% Fat	3 g
CALCIUM	146 mg
IRON	4 mg
SODIUM	46 mg

In a medium-size nonreactive saucepan combine the cranberry juice, sugar, lemon peel, orange peel, vanilla, cinnamon stick and cloves, and bring to a boil over medium-high heat. Reduce the heat to low and simmer the mixture for 5 minutes. Add the pear halves and simmer for another 15 minutes, turning occasionally. Remove the pan from the heat; remove and discard the cinnamon stick and cloves. Transfer the pear halves and poaching liquid to a small bowl and set aside to cool to room temperature, basting the pears often with the liquid if they are not completely immersed. Refrigerate the pears for at least 30 minutes, or until well chilled. To serve, spoon 1/4 cup of yogurt over each pear half and sprinkle with sesame seeds.   Makes 2 servings

RYE-CHEESE CRACKERS

Instead of buying a package of fatty, highly salted snacks, keep these low-calorie crackers on hand to assuage the craving for something crunchy.

1 cup unbleached all-purpose flour, approximately	1 tablespoon unsalted butter or margarine, well chilled
1/2 cup light rye flour	1 1/2 teaspoons caraway seeds
1/2 teaspoon salt	2 tablespoons grated Parmesan

CALORIES per serving	85
77% Carbohydrate	15 g
12% Protein	2 g
18% Fat	2 g
CALCIUM	21 mg
IRON	1 mg
SODIUM	129 mg

In a medium-size bowl stir together 1 cup of the all-purpose flour, the rye flour and salt. Cut the butter into pieces, then with your fingers work it into the dry ingredients until the mixture resembles coarse meal. Add the caraway seeds and 1/2 cup of cold water and stir until the dough begins to gather into a mass, then form it into a ball with your hands. Flatten the dough into a disk, wrap it in plastic wrap and let it rest at room temperature for 30 minutes.

Preheat the oven to 300° F. Lightly flour the work surface and a rolling pin. Cut the dough in half and roll out half to a 1/16-inch-thick rectangle. Using small (2-inch) cookie cutters, cut out about 30 crackers, cutting them as close together as possible. (Do not reroll any excess dough; it will be tough when baked.) Transfer the crackers to a baking sheet and repeat with the remaining dough. Sprinkle the crackers with Parmesan and bake for 12 minutes, or until crisp and lightly browned. Transfer the crackers to racks to cool, then store in an airtight container for up to 1 week.   Makes 10 servings

Note: Instead of cutting the dough with cookie cutters, you can use a ruler and a sharp knife to cut it into 2 1/2-inch squares.

RICE CAKES WITH VEGETABLE-CHEESE SPREAD

An herbed ricotta and vegetable topping is a fine nutritional complement to crisp rice cakes, which are made from whole grains with no added fat.

CALORIES per serving	86
63% Carbohydrate	13 g
19% Protein	4 g
18% Fat	2 g
CALCIUM	75 mg
IRON	1 mg
SODIUM	45 mg

1/2 cup part skim-milk ricotta cheese

2 cups grated carrots

3/4 cup finely chopped red bell pepper

1/4 cup finely chopped celery

3 tablespoons chopped scallion

2 tablespoons chopped fresh parsley

1/2 teaspoon chopped fresh thyme, or 1/4 teaspoon dried thyme

1 tablespoon lemon juice

1/4 teaspoon grated lemon peel

6 rice cakes

Purée the ricotta in a food processor or blender until completely smooth. Stir in the chopped vegetables, herbs, lemon juice and lemon peel, and stir until well combined. Spread 1/2 cup of the mixture on each rice cake and serve.

Makes 6 servings

RYE-CRACKED WHEAT FLATBREAD

Packaged crackers may derive up to 60 percent of their calories from highly saturated fats such as lard, palm kernel oil and coconut oil. However, most of the cooking oils sold for home use are low in saturated fats. Sunflower and safflower oils are among the lowest.

CALORIES per serving	100
72% Carbohydrate	18 g
11% Protein	3 g
17% Fat	2 g
CALCIUM	12 mg
IRON	1 mg
SODIUM	77 mg

3 tablespoons cracked wheat

3/4 teaspoon dry yeast

1 1/2 tablespoon brown sugar

1/2 cup unbleached all-purpose flour, approximately

3/4 cup rye flour

2 teaspoons nonfat dry milk

1 tablespoon vegetable oil

1 large egg white

1/4 teaspoon salt

Place the cracked wheat in a small bowl, add 1/4 cup boiling water and set aside to soak for 5 minutes. Combine the yeast, sugar and 1/4 cup warm water (105-115° F) in a small bowl and set aside for 5 minutes.

Combine 1/2 cup of all-purpose flour, the rye flour, nonfat dry milk, 2 teaspoons of oil, the egg white, cracked wheat and 1/8 teaspoon of salt in the container of a food processor. Start the machine, then pour in the yeast mixture through the feed tube. Process for 40 seconds; the dough should form a ball. Transfer to a medium-size bowl, cover with a kitchen towel and set aside in a warm place to rise for 50 minutes, or until doubled in bulk.

Preheat the oven to 400° F. Lightly flour the work surface. Punch down the dough and roll it out to a 10 x 16-inch rectangle. Cut the dough in half to form two 5 x 16-inch rectangles, transfer one to a baking sheet and prick it all over with a fork. Cut the dough vertically into 6 equal strips, then cut each strip diagonally to form 12 long triangles. Separate the triangles slightly. Place the second sheet of dough on another baking sheet and cut it in the same fashion. Bake the flatbreads in the center of the oven for 8 to 10 minutes, or until golden. With a pastry brush, brush the hot flatbreads with the remaining oil, then sprinkle them with the remaining salt. Transfer the flatbreads to a rack to cool, or serve them warm.

Makes 8 servings (24 flatbreads)

Note: The cooled flatbreads should be stored in an airtight container; they will keep for up to 1 week. Reheat them briefly in a warm oven before serving.

L *ittle changes can add up: If you drink three cups of coffee a day and have a teaspoon of cream in each, giving up the cream — with no other changes in your diet — would cause you to lose four pounds in a year. Or, if you gave up a tablespoon of butter every day for a year, you would lose 10 pounds.*

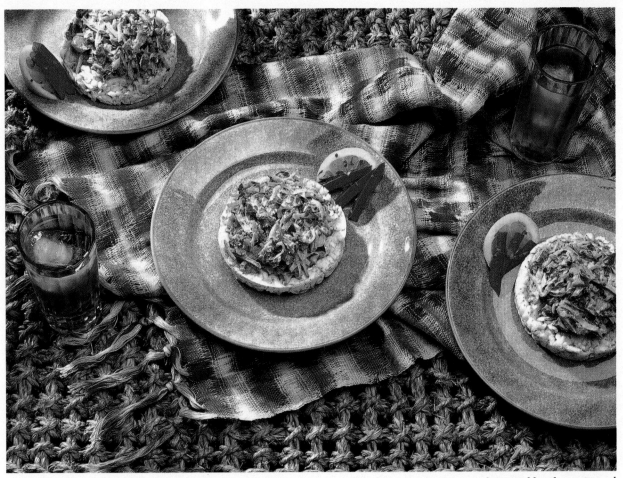

Rice Cakes with Vegetable-Cheese Spread

WHOLE-WHEAT CRANBERRY MUFFINS

Whipped margarine is lower in calories and fat than stick margarine because air is beaten into it. Low-calorie imitation or diet margarines replace some of their oil with water, but they do not work well in baking.

Vegetable cooking spray
  (optional)
1 cup whole-wheat flour
1/2 cup unbleached
  all-purpose flour
2 teaspoons baking powder
1/2 teapoon ground cinnamon
Pinch of salt

1/2 cup skim milk
1/4 cup whipped margarine,
  melted and cooled
1/4 cup honey
1 large egg, lightly beaten
1 1/2 cups cranberries,
  coarsely chopped

CALORIES per muffin	142
65% Carbohydrate	23 g
9% Protein	3 g
26% Fat	4 g
CALCIUM	69 mg
IRON	1 mg
SODIUM	141 mg

Preheat the oven to 400° F. Lighly spray 10 muffin tin cups with cooking spray or line them with paper liners; set aside. In a large bowl stir together the flours, baking powder, cinnamon and salt. In a small bowl stir together the milk, margarine, honey and egg. Add the milk mixture to the dry ingredients and stir vigorously for 30 seconds. Stir in the cranberries. Divide the batter among the muffin cups and bake for 30 minutes, or until the tops are golden and a toothpick inserted in a muffin comes out clean.   Makes 10 muffins

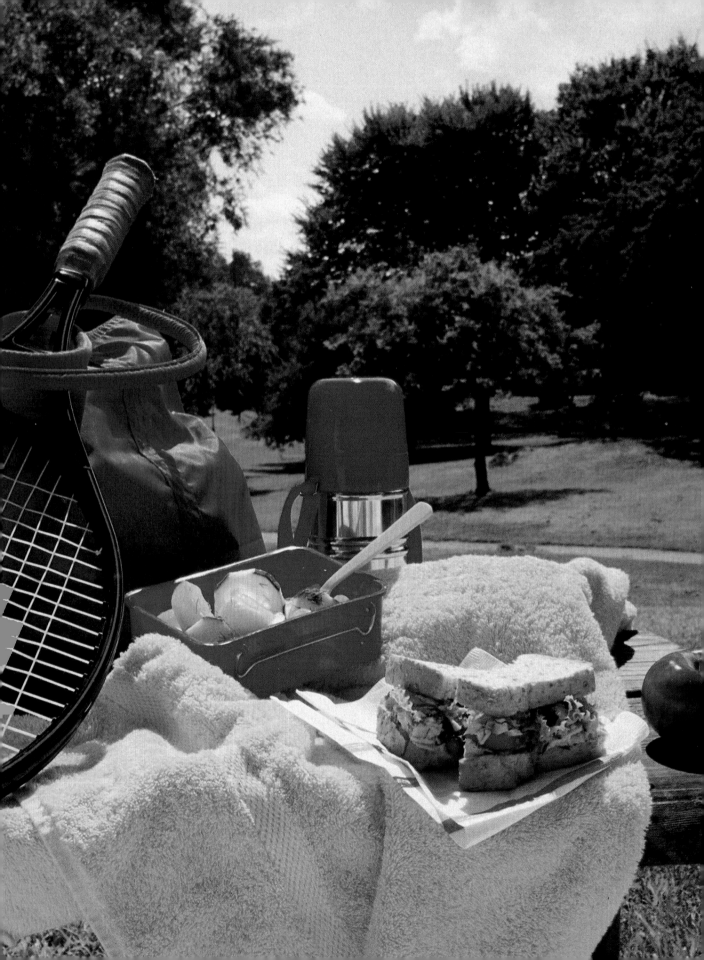

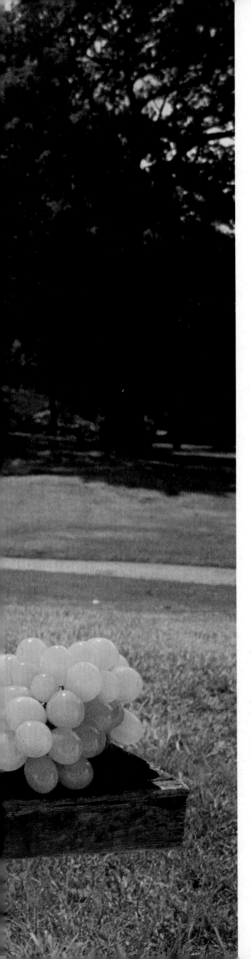

CHAPTER THREE

Lunch

Avoiding the unwanted calories in sandwiches and at salad bars

For the midday meal, many weight-conscious people face the problem of choosing foods from a cafeteria, delicatessen or fast-food restaurant where they have little or no control over the ingredients in a dish or its preparation. Consider sandwiches: Those made in a deli are typically packed with cold cuts that derive up to 80 percent of their calories from fat. Bologna, for example, has 90 calories per ounce, and a bologna sandwich may contain five to 10 ounces of meat. Such a sandwich might be served with a side order of coleslaw or potato salad, both of which generally contain large amounts of high-fat mayonnaise. In fact, dressings and side dishes accompanying a sandwich can be the source of hidden calories at lunch. A three-ounce hamburger in a bun has a fairly modest 300 to 350 calories. But if the burger is topped with a mayonnaise-based sauce, condiments or cheese, or if it is served with French fries or deep-fried onion rings, the calories you consume for your lunch may be more than double those of a plain hamburger.

In their quest for a lighter, more nutritious lunch, growing numbers of Americans are turning to salad bars. Despite their healthy image, however, many salad bars offer foods full of unexpected calories. Alongside low-calorie vegetables and fruits, you are likely to find bacon bits, diced ham, olives, avocados and cheese — all of which would add a large amount of calories to a lowfat meal. The oil-based dressings you can add to salad-bar ingredients can raise the calorie count by 50-100 calories per spoonful. A university study that compared students who ate a salad-bar lunch with those who ate a cafeteria hot meal found that the salad-bar patrons consumed more calories than the other group and that a greater percentage of their calories came from fat.

The best weight-control strategy for lunch is to make your own meal, which will also ensure its nutritional value. You can draw on a variety of foods — fruits, vegetables, lowfat cheeses and yogurt, fish, pasta, grains, legumes and poultry — that will fill you up without adding excess calories. Instead of having an overstuffed processed-meat sandwich, for example, use skinless turkey breast or chicken, both of which have about half the calories of bologna or salami. Tuna packed in water, not in oil, is also a good choice. You can reduce the fat content of a sandwich even further by supplementing a small amount of meat with vegetables, as in the vegetable-and-chicken sandwich on page 98. And instead of adding butter, margarine or mayonnaise, substitute lowfat yogurt, mustard or horseradish.

Salads make excellent low-calorie, nutrient-rich lunches. Instead of the standard mixed green salad, you can use denser, more filling ingredients, as in the halibut salad on page 92, which combines fish with asparagus, oranges and a sweet potato, or the green salad with chicken and mangoes on page 87. The oil in conventional dressings can turn any salad into a high-calorie dish, so dress your salad with vinegar and herbs, lemon juice or lowfat yogurt, and keep the amount of oil to a teaspoon or less per serving. A good example is the dressing for the apple, fennel and pasta salad on page 98, which uses balsamic vinegar and oil in proportions that are almost the reverse of many oil-heavy dressings served in restaurants and at salad bars.

One of the best weight-conscious choices for lunchtime is soup, which has a lower caloric density than most solid foods and which tends to take longer to eat. Research indicates that people who eat soup tend to feel full before they have consumed many calories. In one study, subjects who were served low-calorie tomato soup reported feeling full on the same amount of soup as subjects who ate a higher-calorie soup. Yet the first group consumed approximately one tenth of the calories consumed by the second group. The curried vegetable soup on page 91 and scallop soup on page 88 use lowfat ingredients that are substantial enough to keep you from overeating, and they are also low in sodium, which is often added to commercial canned soups in the form of salt and monosodium glutamate (MSG).

Skipping lunch is one weight-control strategy you should not adopt.

Choosing a Beverage

Even if you are conscientious about what you eat at lunchtime, your attempt to control your weight may be foiled if you do not pay equal attention to what you drink. The following guidelines point out the calorie content of various beverages and their effect on your diet.

◆ Water is one of the best thirst-quenchers, whether you drink it in the form of club soda, seltzer, mineral water or plain tap water. It relieves your thirst as effectively as other types of beverages, or even better, and it has no calories. Club sodas and many mineral waters generally contain sodium, but salt-free varieties are available.

◆ Soft drinks are among the worst drinks for those seeking to control their weight. Nondiet soft drinks typically contain 140-150 calories per 12-ounce can, and 99 percent of these calories may come from sugar. Diet soft drinks that contain the artificial sweetener aspartame have no calories, but they may have unwanted side effects for sensitive people.

◆ Fruit juices are often good sources of vitamins and minerals, but they contain a significant amount of calories. An eight-ounce glass of orange juice, for example, has about 110 calories, and a glass of canned pineapple juice has 140. You can retain much of the taste of juice while reducing its calories by diluting it with seltzer.

◆ Alcoholic beverages tend to be high in calories and low in nutrients. There are about 150 calories in a 12-ounce bottle of beer. Light beers contain about 100, and a six-ounce glass of wine contains about 160. Hard liquors are even more concentrated: One shot (1 1/2 ounces) of 80-proof gin, vodka or whiskey contains 95 calories, and if you add a mixer, you may consume more than 200 calories. There is also some indication that the alcohol in one or two drinks can increase your appetite. Therefore, if you do drink alcoholic beverages, restrict your intake and drink during a meal rather than beforehand.

◆ Coffee and tea usually have fewer than five calories per cup. But when you add whole milk, cream or a nondairy creamer — which is mostly oil — you are adding some 25 calories per serving. And presweetened teas or coffees contain many more calories. The caffeine in coffee and tea can also cause such side effects as irritability, headaches and nervousness when consumed in excess, so it is a good idea to drink no more than two cups a day.

Because of work-related pressures and because lunch breaks can be short, you may be tempted not to eat, and one recent survey shows that more and more Americans do that regularly. But not eating in the middle of the day may encourage binging or overeating in the afternoon and evening. Lunch skippers are likely to resort to eating a succession of snacks like pretzels, potato chips, cookies, candy bars and other foods that are typically high in sugar and sodium, refined flours and saturated fats. Having lunch not only helps you avoid overeating later, but boosts your energy level during the afternoon. If you want a snack in midafternoon, choose one from those recommended on pages 78-79. You can also make one of the recipes on pages 102-107 as a satisfying alternative to more conventional snacks.

Controlling Cravings

The impulse to eat food that you want but do not need can be troublesome when you follow a reduced-calorie diet. Even scientists who have studied the subject cannot explain why people have sudden and sometimes uncontrollable urges for certain foods or taste sensations. Researchers do know, however, that many cravings have psychological, rather than physical, causes.

Your appetite for food is a combination of your body chemistry, the functioning of your senses and the psychological connotations a particular food may have for you. The secretion of the female hormone progesterone, for example, may account for the cravings women experience during menstruation and pregnancy. One study found that women consume 30 percent more carbohydrates during menstruation than they do during the rest of their menstrual cycle.

Opinion is divided on a possible link between carbohydrate cravings and a brain substance called serotonin. Some scientists suspect that eating carbohydrates helps certain people to overcome anxiety or depression. Ongoing research may clarify whether a person's carbohydrate consumption prompts the brain to make enough serotonin to elevate his or her mood.

Why certain tastes have special appeal to people is not well understood. A craving for sugar may be genetic — in studies of infants, a widespread preference for sweets has been observed. The same may be true of salt, which, after sugar, is the most commonly used food additive. But some reasearchers think that cravings are more a matter of eating habits than of taste appeal.

Examining your own emotional attachments to food may be the best approach to controlling those cravings that are stress-related. For example, if you tend to eat a candy bar, a cookie or another form of sweets when a stressful situation confronts you, it may be that a parent always gave you candy to calm you down when you were upset as a child. Once you have recognized the origin of a bad habit, you may be able to break it.

One of the best ways to handle cravings is to monitor and control your snacks, since most weight-loss plans minimize between-meal eating. The chart opposite shows the wide range of snacks that are recommended. If you consume an afternoon snack at your office, choose items listed in the "excellent" and "acceptable" categories, rather than those from a bakery or candy counter.

Here are some other diet-oriented strategies:

● Identify the specific food you crave. Do not simply eat whatever is available until you feel full.

● Try to satisfy a craving for sweets with a piece of fruit, a glass of fruit juice or a low-sugar cookie. A medium-size apple has 80-90 calories; a typical chewy, chocolaty candy bar has 250.

● Drink a glass of low-salt tomato or other vegetable juice to satisfy a salt craving. Lightly salted, air-popped popcorn is a good alternative to heavily salted pretzels and chips.

● Eat foods high in fiber and complex carbohydrates before you indulge in a less wholesome food you crave. A slice or two of whole-grain bread or a plate of raw vegetables will help fill you up and may distract your attention from sugary or salty snacks.

HOW SNACKS STACK UP

Eating between meals can be an effective hunger-controlling element in a weight-control plan. But fatty snacks violate the basic tenets of a low-calorie diet. The examples below, grouped according to fat content, show what snacks are best.

EXCELLENT

cottage cheese (1%)
fresh fruit
lowfat plain yogurt with fruit
plain bagel
plain breadsticks
raw vegetables
rice cake
unbuttered popcorn, air-popped
unsweetened cereal with skim milk
whole-wheat bread with all-fruit preserves

ACCEPTABLE

bagel with melted part skim-milk mozzarella
corn bread
dried fruit
dry roasted nuts, no salt
flavored gelatin with fresh fruit
flavored ices
gingersnaps
lowfat vanilla yogurt
pretzels
ricotta cheese and rye crackers
white bread toast with jam

NOT RECOMMENDED

brownie
candy bar
chocolate chip cookies
chocolate pudding
cream-filled doughnut
croissant with butter
Danish pastry
éclair
ice cream
milk shake
potato chips

Body Toning

As you are losing weight, exercises to shape and tone your muscles will help you develop an esthetically pleasing physique. Firm, strong muscles also contribute to weight loss; as your muscle mass increases with strength training, your calorie expenditure is accelerated. Even at rest, muscle tissue burns more calories than fat tissue.

As a result of inactivity, however, many people lose muscle mass as they gain fat around their waist and thighs. Weakened musculature also affects posture. When stomach muscles sag, they may contribute to excessive curvature of the back or spine, forcing the back to hold up more than its share of body weight and resulting in lower back pain.

The exercises on these two pages can restore your body's pleasing proportions, make your shoulders appear broader and draw them back, expand your chest, improve your posture and strengthen your abdominals to reduce and prevent lower back pain. Perform these exercises three days a week, with a day of rest between days of exercise. Start with a five-pound hand weight and perform each exercise until you can complete three sets of 10 repetitions. As you become stronger and more experienced, you can increase the load of the weights.

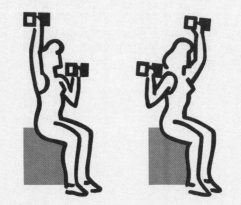

1. Strengthen your shoulders and upper arms by alternately pressing and lowering dumbbells with your palms facing forward.

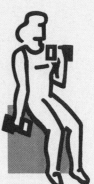

2. To condition your biceps, alternately raise and lower the dumbbells from your hips to your shoulders with your palms up.

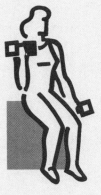

3. To condition the back of your upper arms and your upper back muscles, hold the upper end of a dumbbell with both hands over your head. Lower the weight behind your head, then press it to the starting position.

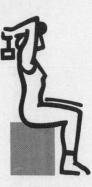

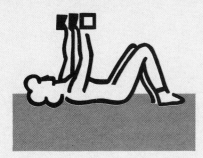

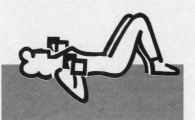

4. Lie on your back with your feet flat on an exercise bench. Face your palms forward and press the dumbbells directly over your shoulders. Lower the weights to slightly below your shoulders.

5. On an exercise bench, raise the dumbbells directly over your shoulders and keep your elbows slightly bent. Lower the dumbbells outward, and then return to strengthen the chest.

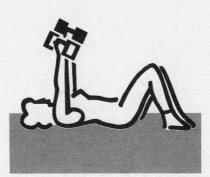

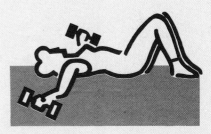

6. To condition your back and shoulder muscles, grasp two dumbbells and sit on a bench. Bend at the waist so that the dumbbells hang near the ankles. Slowly raise the dumbbells sideways to about shoulder level and then lower again.

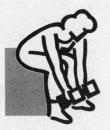

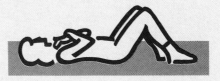

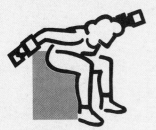

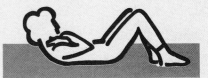

7. Perform bent-knee curls to strengthen the abdominals. Lie on your back with your feet flat on the floor and your hands across your chest. Curl only your head and upper back off the floor and return to starting position.

SOLE IN PARCHMENT ▼

Fish contains the same quality protein as red meat, but with a much lower calorie count per pound. This cooking method keeps even lean fish moist.

CALORIES per serving	179
49% Carbohydrate	22 g
28% Protein	13 g
23% Fat	5 g
CALCIUM	40 mg
IRON	2 mg
SODIUM	255 mg

4 teaspoons butter
1/3 cup sliced scallions
2 teaspoons lemon juice
1 garlic clove, minced
1/2 teaspoon caraway seeds
1/4 teaspoon salt
1/8 teaspoon paprika
Black pepper

Dash of hot pepper sauce
1/2 pound fillet of sole,
   cut into 4 equal pieces
6 small unpeeled red potatoes
   (about 14 ounces total weight),
   boiled and sliced 1/4 inch thick
6 ounces snow peas, trimmed
   and blanched

Preheat the oven to 350° F. Melt the butter in a small saucepan over low heat. Stir in the scallions, lemon juice, garlic, caraway seeds, salt, paprika, pepper and hot pepper sauce. Cook for 2 to 3 minutes, or until fragrant; set aside.

Cut four 12-inch circles of parchment paper or heavy-duty aluminum foil. Place a portion of sole on one side of each circle and divide the potatoes and snow peas among the four portions. Spoon the butter mixture over the fish and vegetables, then fold the other side of the parchment over the fish and vegetables and firmly crimp the edges to seal them. Place the packets on a baking sheet and bake for 12 minutes, or until the fish flakes when tested with a knife. Place each parchment packet on a plate and open the packets just before serving.   Makes 4 servings

PASTA AND CAULIFLOWER WITH SESAME SAUCE

The vegetables tossed with the pasta in this recipe make for generous portions while adding only 30 calories per serving. The cauliflower and bell pepper provide twice your daily requirement of vitamin C.

4 cups cauliflower florets
1/2 cup plain lowfat yogurt
1 tablespoon plus 1 teaspoon
   Oriental sesame oil
1 tablespoon toasted
   sesame seeds
1 teaspoon lemon juice

1 large red bell pepper, cut into
   1/4-inch-wide strips
1/2 pound spinach rotelle
   (spiral pasta)
1/2 teaspoon salt
1/4 teaspoon red pepper flakes
Black pepper

CALORIES per serving	320
60% Carbohydrate	49 g
15% Protein	12 g
25% Fat	9 g
CALCIUM	107 mg
IRON	3 mg
SODIUM	313 mg

Bring a large saucepan of water to a boil. Add the cauliflower and cook it for 10 minutes, or until fork-tender. (If you prefer crisper cauliflower, cook it for 8 minutes.) Meanwhile, for the dressing, in a large bowl whisk together the yogurt, oil, sesame seeds and lemon juice. Add the bell pepper strips and toss to coat; set aside.

Reserving the boiling water, use a slotted spoon to transfer the cauliflower to a colander; cool under cold running water and drain. Cook the pasta in the boiling water for 8 minutes, or according to package directions until al dente; cool under cold water and drain thoroughly. Add the pasta and cauliflower to the dressing and toss until well combined. Add the salt and red pepper flakes, and black pepper to taste, and toss again.   Makes 4 servings

Sole in Parchment ▷

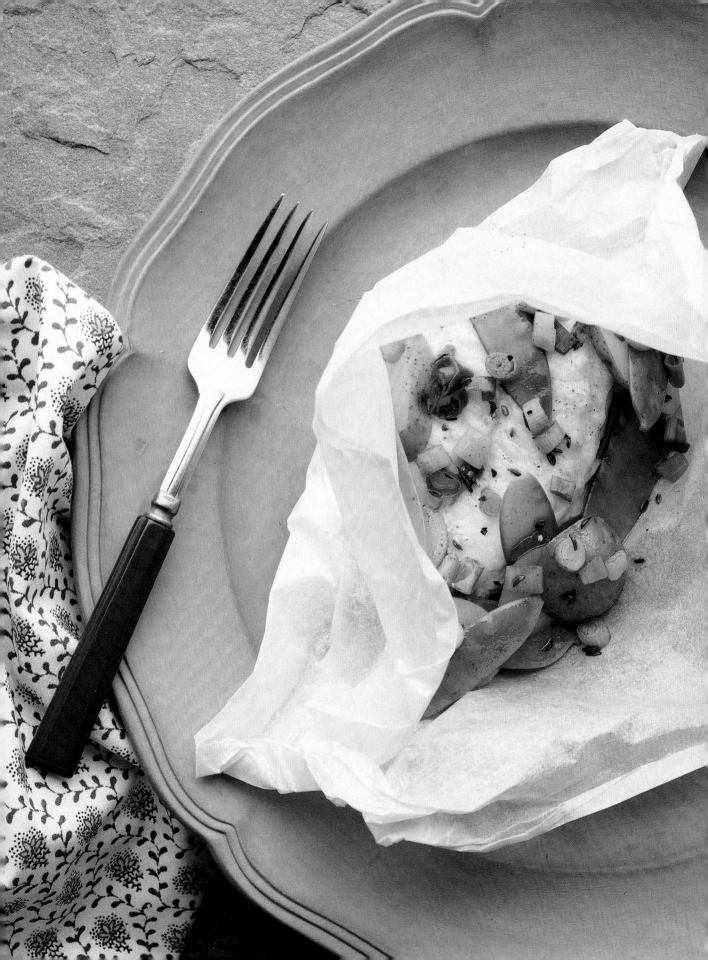

TOMATO AND BASIL TART WITH CHÈVRE ▼

The paper-thin pastry leaves called phyllo are usually brushed with melted butter before baking, but they work well here without the added fat.

CALORIES per serving	271
50% Carbohydrate	36 g
21% Protein	15 g
29% Fat	9 g
CALCIUM	155 mg
IRON	5 mg
SODIUM	392 mg

1 1/2 pounds fresh plum tomatoes
2 tablespoons low-sodium chicken stock
1 cup chopped onion
3 cups chopped fresh spinach
2 cups diced summer squash
2 cups chopped fresh mushrooms
1/4 cup chopped fresh basil
1 garlic clove, minced
1/4 teaspoon salt
1/4 teaspoon pepper
4 sheets phyllo dough
3 large eggs
1/4 cup plain lowfat yogurt
Pinch of grated nutmeg
2 ounces chèvre (mild goat cheese), cut into small pieces
Vegetable cooking spray

Preheat the oven to 350° F. Peel, seed and chop the tomatoes and set aside in a colander to drain. Heat the stock in a large nonstick skillet over high heat. Add the onion, reduce the heat to medium and cook, stirring occasionally, for 5 minutes. Add the tomatoes, spinach, squash, mushrooms, basil, garlic, salt and pepper, and cover the skillet. Cook, stirring occasionally, for another 5 minutes. Uncover the skillet and cook, stirring, for 2 minutes more, or until the spinach is wilted. Remove the skillet from the heat and set aside to cool.

Separate the phyllo. Fit one sheet into an 8 1/2-inch tart pan, folding in the edges to leave a 2-inch overhang. Repeat with the remaining phyllo. In a small bowl whisk together the eggs, yogurt and nutmeg. Using a slotted spoon to drain the vegetables well, spoon them into the tart pan. Pour the egg mixture over the vegetables and dot with chèvre. Roll and crimp the edges of the phyllo to form a rim and spray it with cooking spray. Bake the tart for 40 minutes, or until the filling is set and the pastry is light golden. Let the tart stand for 5 minutes, then cut it in quarters and serve. Makes 4 servings

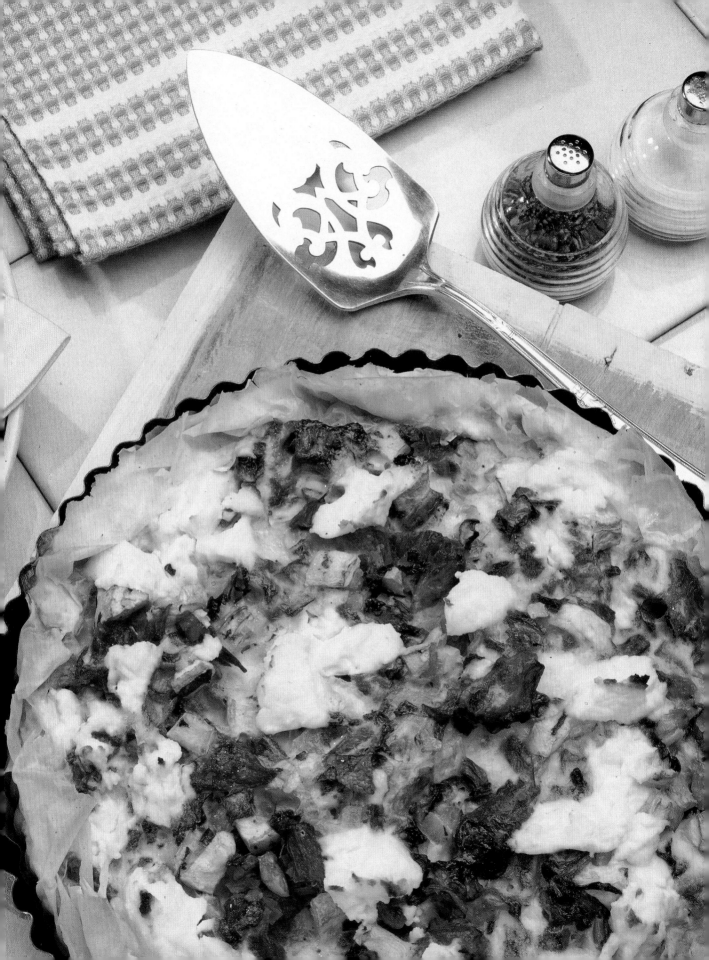

CALORIES per serving	272
65% Carbohydrate	43 g
11% Protein	7 g
24% Fat	7 g
CALCIUM	146 mg
IRON	2 mg
SODIUM	369 mg

STRAWBERRY SHORTCAKE WITH YOGURT BISCUITS

You can treat yourself to a luxurious dessert and still keep calories low with the right ingredient substitutions. Margarine and yogurt replace butter in these biscuits, and lowfat ricotta, instead of whipped cream, tops them.

1 pint fresh strawberries
4 teaspoons brown sugar
1/4 cup part skim-milk ricotta
1 tablespoon lemon juice
1 1/2 teaspoons grated lemon peel
1 1/4 cups unbleached
   all-purpose flour, approximately

1 teaspoon baking powder
1/4 teaspoon baking soda
1/4 teaspoon salt
1/4 teaspoon cinnamon
2 1/2 tablespoons whipped
   margarine, well chilled
1/4 cup plain lowfat yogurt

Wash, hull and slice the strawberries and toss them with 2 teaspoons of sugar in a small bowl. For the ricotta cream, in another small bowl mix together the ricotta, lemon juice, lemon peel and remaining sugar; set aside.

Preheat the oven to 450° F. In a large bowl stir together 1 1/4 cups of flour, the baking powder, baking soda, salt and cinnamon. Using a pastry blender or 2 knives, cut in the margarine until the mixture resembles coarse crumbs. Add the yogurt and 1/4 cup of cold water and stir briefly, then form the dough into a ball with your hands. On a lightly floured surface, knead the dough a few times, then roll it out to a 1/2-inch thickness. Using a 2 1/2-inch biscuit cutter, cut out 8 biscuits. Place them on a baking sheet and bake for 10 to 12 minutes, or until golden. Split the biscuits and place 2 of the bottom halves on each of 4 plates. Top each half with 2 tablespoons of strawberries and 1 1/2 teaspoons of ricotta cream and cover with the biscuit tops.   Makes 4 servings

*H*eading for the salad bar is a good lunchtime instinct if you are trying to lose weight, but choose carefully: Dressings and sauces can sabotage a low-calorie meal. A half-cup of cooked elbow macaroni has just 77 calories, but the same amount of macaroni salad has about 215 calories. A half-cup serving of water-packed tuna has 127 calories, while an equal amount of tuna salad with mayonnaise has 175 calories.

GRILLED VEGETABLE-CHEDDAR SANDWICH ▼

This sandwich is reminiscent of a cheeseburger — with less than half the fat.

Vegetable cooking spray
One 6-ounce eggplant
2 cups sliced mushrooms
1/4 pound Cheddar cheese, grated
1 cup thinly sliced scallions

2 cups bean sprouts
3 cups lettuce, torn into
   bite-size pieces
8 slices whole-grain bread
2 tablespoons Dijon-style mustard

Preheat the oven to 350° F. Spray a baking sheet with cooking spray. Cut the eggplant into 1/4-inch-thick slices, lay them on the baking sheet and bake for 10 minutes, or until tender; set aside to cool. Meanwhile, place the mushrooms in a medium-size skillet with 2 tablespoons of water and sauté over medium heat for 3 to 5 minutes, or until softened. Divide the cheese, mushrooms, scallions, sprouts and lettuce among 4 slices of bread and top with the eggplant slices. Spread the 4 remaining slices of bread with mustard, place them on the sandwiches and press them firmly with your hand so they hold together during cooking. Spray a large nonstick skillet with cooking spray and heat it over medium-high heat. Place a sandwich cheese-side down in the skillet and heat it, pressing it with a metal spatula, for 3 to 4 minutes, or until the cheese is melted, then turn the sandwich and cook for another 3 to 4 minutes, or until the bread is lightly browned.   Makes 4 servings

CALORIES per serving	227
55% Carbohydrate	33 g
20% Protein	12 g
25% Fat	7 g
CALCIUM	215 mg
IRON	4 mg
SODIUM	564 mg

GREEN SALAD WITH CHICKEN AND MANGOES

Niacin is found in fatty foods such as beef and peanuts, but you can get half your daily requirement of niacin from the chicken and mangoes in this salad.

CALORIES per serving	326
54% Carbohydrate	47 g
24% Protein	21 g
22% Fat	9 g
CALCIUM	241 mg
IRON	4 mg
SODIUM	236 mg

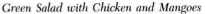

1/2 pound boneless, skinless chicken breast

1/2 cup low-sodium chicken stock

1/4 cup lemon juice

2 tablespoons olive oil

1 teaspoon finely chopped fresh tarragon, or 1/4 teaspoon dried tarragon, crumbled

1/4 teaspoon salt

1/4 teaspoon black pepper

2 heads Romaine lettuce

2 bunches watercress

2 cups diced red bell peppers

1 cup shredded red cabbage

1 cup finely chopped scallions

4 mangoes, peeled and diced

Place the chicken in a small saucepan, add cold water to cover and bring to a boil over medium-high heat. Reduce the heat so that the water simmers and poach the chicken for 5 minutes, or just until cooked through; transfer it to a plate and set aside to cool to room temperature.

For the dressing, in a small bowl whisk together the stock, lemon juice, oil, tarragon, salt and pepper; set aside. Wash the Romaine and watercress. Tear the Romaine into bite-size pieces, trim the watercress and combine the greens in a large bowl. Add the cabbage and scallions and toss well.

Cut the chicken diagonally into thin slices. Whisk the dressing briefly to reblend it. Add the chicken, mangoes and dressing to the salad and toss gently. Divide the salad among 4 plates and serve.   Makes 4 servings

Green Salad with Chicken and Mangoes

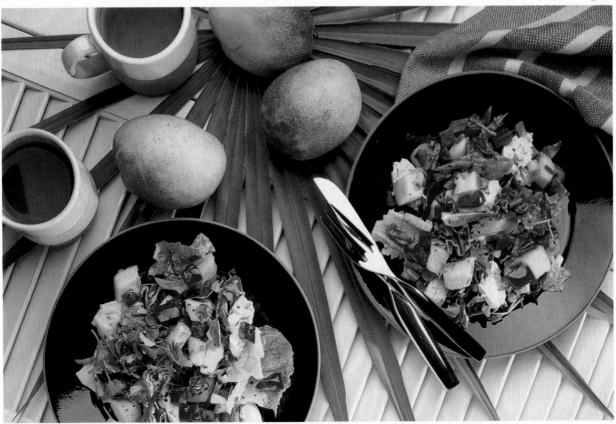

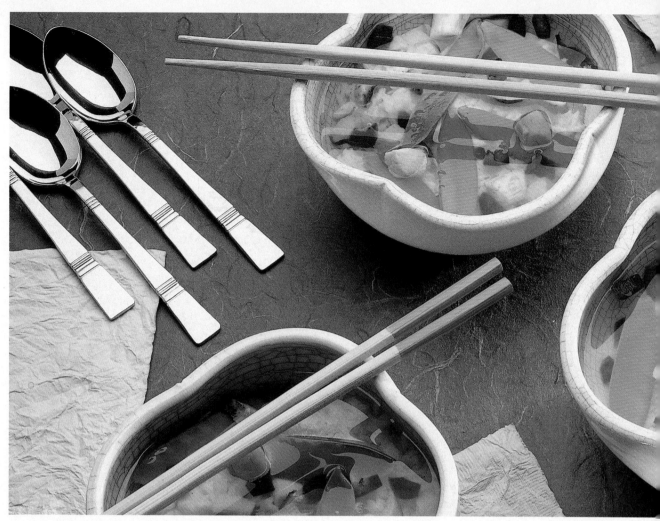

Oriental Scallop Soup

ORIENTAL SCALLOP SOUP ▼

Scallops are lower in fat and cholesterol than most fish and shellfish.

2 teaspoons vegetable oil	1 3/4 cups sliced shiitake
2 ounces bay scallops	mushrooms or white mushrooms
4 cups low-sodium chicken stock	3/4 cup cooked white rice
1 1/2 cups chopped carrots	1/2 cup finely diced red bell pepper
1/3 cup chopped scallions	3 ounces snow peas, trimmed
1 teaspoon minced fresh ginger	1/4 cup sake (Japanese rice wine)

Heat the oil in a medium-size saucepan over medium heat. Add the scallops and sauté for 2 minutes, or until the scallops are opaque and firm; transfer the scallops to a small bowl and set aside. Place the stock, carrots, scallions and ginger in the saucepan, bring to a simmer over medium heat and cook for 15 minutes. Strain the stock into a large bowl and discard the solids. Return the stock to the pan, add the mushrooms and simmer for 2 minutes, or until the mushrooms are soft. Stir in the scallops, rice, bell pepper, snow peas, sake and 1/2 cup of water, and cook for another 3 minutes, or until the soup is heated through. Ladle the soup into 4 bowls and serve.   Makes 4 servings

CALORIES per serving	142
59% Carbohydrate	20 g
23% Protein	7 g
18% Fat	3 g
CALCIUM	50 mg
IRON	3 mg
SODIUM	95 mg

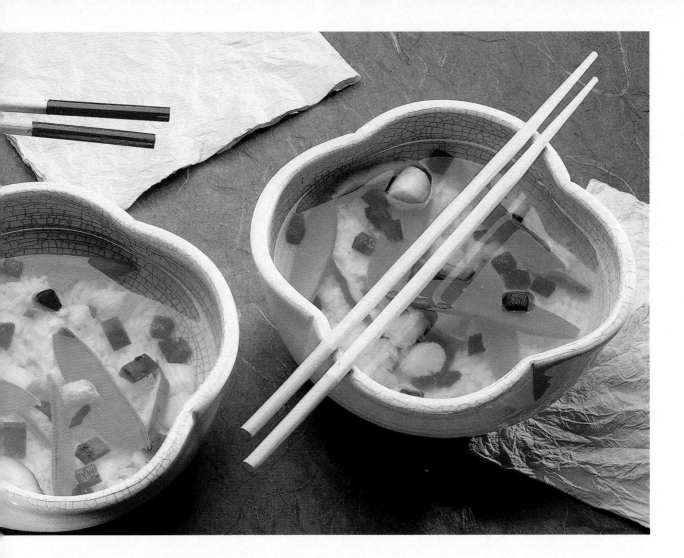

VELVETY VEGETABLE DRINK ▼

You can prepare this drink the day before serving it and chill it overnight.
With a salad and some whole-grain bread, it makes a light lunch.

2 cups low-sodium tomato juice
Small bunch fresh parsley
10 watercress sprigs
1 cup finely chopped carrots
3/4 cup finely chopped celery

3/4 cup finely chopped
 red bell pepper
1/4 cup plain lowfat yogurt
1 teaspoon olive oil,
 preferably extra-virgin

In a medium-size saucepan combine the tomato juice, parsley, watercress, carrots, celery and bell pepper and bring to a boil over medium-high heat. Cover the pan, reduce the heat to low and simmer for 20 minutes, or until the vegetables are soft. Remove the pan from the heat and let the mixture cool slightly. Remove and discard the stems from the parsley and watercress and return the leaves to the saucepan. Transfer the mixture to a blender and process until puréed, then set aside to cool. Transfer the mixture to a pitcher, stir in the yogurt and oil, cover and refrigerate until well chilled. Divide the drink between 2 tall ice-filled glasses and serve.   Makes 2 servings

CALORIES per serving	146
67% Carbohydrate	27 g
15% Protein	6 g
18% Fat	3 g
CALCIUM	200 mg
IRON	6 mg
SODIUM	137 mg

THREE-MELON SALAD WITH
RASPBERRY VINAIGRETTE ▼

The dressing can make or break a low-calorie salad: The vinaigrette, farmer cheese and pecans used here total about 86 calories per serving. A comparable amount of blue cheese dressing has more than 200 calories.

CALORIES per serving	240
59% Carbohydrate	39 g
10% Protein	7 g
31% Fat	9 g
CALCIUM	51 mg
IRON	1 mg
SODIUM	357 mg

3 tablespoons raspberry vinegar, or to taste
1 tablespoon safflower oil
1 tablespoon lemon juice
1/2 teaspoon salt
4 cups 1-inch cantaloupe chunks
3 cups 1-inch honeydew chunks
4 cups watermelon balls or chunks

3 ounces farmer cheese or pot cheese
1/2 cup chopped fresh mint leaves
4 large Romaine lettuce leaves, washed and trimmed
2 tablespoons coarsely chopped pecans

For the dressing, in a small bowl whisk together the vinegar, oil, lemon juice and salt; set aside. Combine the cantaloupe, honeydew and watermelon in a large bowl, add the dressing and toss gently. Cover the bowl and refrigerate for at least 1 hour. Just before serving, crumble the cheese into a small bowl, add the mint and mash with a fork to combine. Line a serving platter with Romaine leaves and mound the melon on it. Sprinkle the cheese over the melon and scatter the pecans on top.   Makes 4 servings

COUSCOUS

Americans typically eat large portions of meat with small side dishes of vegetables and grains. This Moroccan-style meal, like many ethnic dishes, reverses those proportions for a healthier, less caloric lunch.

CALORIES per serving	375
65% Carbohydrate	53 g
14% Protein	12 g
21% Fat	8 g
CALCIUM	54 mg
IRON	2 mg
SODIUM	397 mg

2 tablespoons olive oil
1/2 teaspoon each ground
    cinnamon, cumin and paprika
2 or 3 saffron threads, crumbled
1 medium-size onion, sliced
3/4 cup sliced carrots
1 cup diced parsnips
10 dried apricot halves

1 small chicken thigh, skinned
1 cup canned plum tomatoes,
    drained and diced
1 1/4 cups instant couscous
1/2 teaspoon salt
Black pepper
2 tablespoons chopped
    fresh coriander

Heat the oil in a large heavy-gauge saucepan over medium heat. Add the cinnamon, cumin, paprika and saffron, and cook, stirring, for 2 minutes, or until fragrant. Add the onion, carrots, parsnips, apricots and chicken, and sauté, turning the chicken occasionally, for 5 minutes. Add the tomatoes and 4 1/2 cups of water and bring to a boil over medium-high heat. Reduce the heat to low, cover the pan and simmer the mixture for 30 minutes.

Remove the pan from the heat. Remove the chicken, bone it and cut the meat into thin strips; set aside. Stir the couscous into the pan, cover and set aside for 5 minutes. Add the salt, and pepper to taste, scatter the chicken strips over the couscous and sprinkle with coriander.   Makes 4 servings

CURRIED VEGETABLE SOUP ▼

Puréeing some of the vegetables from the soup and adding just a half-cup of lowfat milk makes this a creamy soup without using a drop of cream.

2 tablespoons whipped margarine
1 cup chopped onion
1 cup diced carrots
1 cup diced celery
1 garlic clove, minced
1 tablespoon curry powder
One 28-ounce can plum tomatoes
3 cups cooked split peas
    (6 ounces dried)

2 cups frozen corn kernels
1/2 teaspoon salt
1/2 teaspoon pepper
1/2 cup lowfat milk (2%)
2 cups shredded kale or other leafy
    greens (about 2 1/2 ounces)
1/4 cup chopped fresh coriander
1 ounce low-sodium sesame
    crackers (8 crackers)

Melt the margarine in a large saucepan over medium heat. Add the onion, carrots, celery and garlic, and cook, stirring, for 5 minutes. Add the tomatoes and their liquid and 2 cups of water and bring to a boil over medium-high heat, breaking up the tomatoes with the edge of a spoon. Reduce the heat to low and simmer the soup for 20 minutes. Add the split peas, corn, salt and pepper, and cook for 15 minutes. Using a slotted spoon, transfer three fourths of the vegetables to a food processor or blender and purée, then return the purée to the saucepan. Stir in the milk and cook until heated through. Just before serving, add the kale and stir just until wilted. Ladle the soup into 4 bowls, sprinkle with coriander and serve with the crackers.   Makes 4 servings

CALORIES per serving	265
64% Carbohydrate	45 g
18% Protein	12 g
18% Fat	6 g
CALCIUM	131 mg
IRON	4 mg
SODIUM	483 mg

TAMPA BAY HALIBUT SALAD

The fat content of fish varies greatly; halibut is relatively lean. Furthermore, the fat in fish is good for you in moderation because it contains omega-3 fatty acids, which may help prevent heart disease. In a study reported in the New England Journal of Medicine, *eating 3 ounces of fish per week was associated with a 30 percent reduction in the risk of heart disease.*

1 large sweet potato (about 10 ounces)	1/4 cup chopped shallots
1 1/2 pounds asparagus	4 teaspoons olive oil
1/2 pound 1-inch-thick boneless halibut steak	1 tablespoon rice-wine vinegar
2 navel oranges	1 teaspoon Dijon-style mustard
1/2 cup freshly squeezed orange juice	1/4 teaspoon salt
	8 large Romaine lettuce leaves, washed and trimmed
	4 slices raisin bread

Bring a small saucepan of water to a boil. Wash and trim the sweet potato; do not peel it. Cut the potato into 1-inch chunks and cook it for 20 minutes, or until it is tender. Meanwhile, bring a large pot of water to a boil. Trim the asparagus, cut it into 1-inch pieces and cook it for 5 to 7 minutes, or until it is crisp-tender. Drain, cool under cold water and set aside to drain again. When the potato is done, drain and set aside to cool.

Preheat the oven to 350° F. Rinse and pat dry the halibut, place it in a small baking pan and bake it for 10 minutes, or until the fish flakes when tested with a fork; set aside to cool. Meanwhile, peel and section the oranges and remove the membranes; set aside. For the dressing, in a small bowl stir together the orange juice, shallots, oil, vinegar, mustard and salt. In a large bowl combine the potato, asparagus, halibut and oranges. Add the dressing and toss gently, breaking up the fish as little as possible. Cover the bowl and refrigerate the salad for 3 to 4 hours, tossing it twice while it is chilling.

To serve, line 4 plates with Romaine and mound the halibut salad on top. Toast the bread and serve it with the salad. Makes 4 servings

CALORIES per serving	305
57% Carbohydrate	45 g
24% Protein	19 g
19% Fat	7 g
CALCIUM	113 mg
IRON	3 mg
SODIUM	307 mg

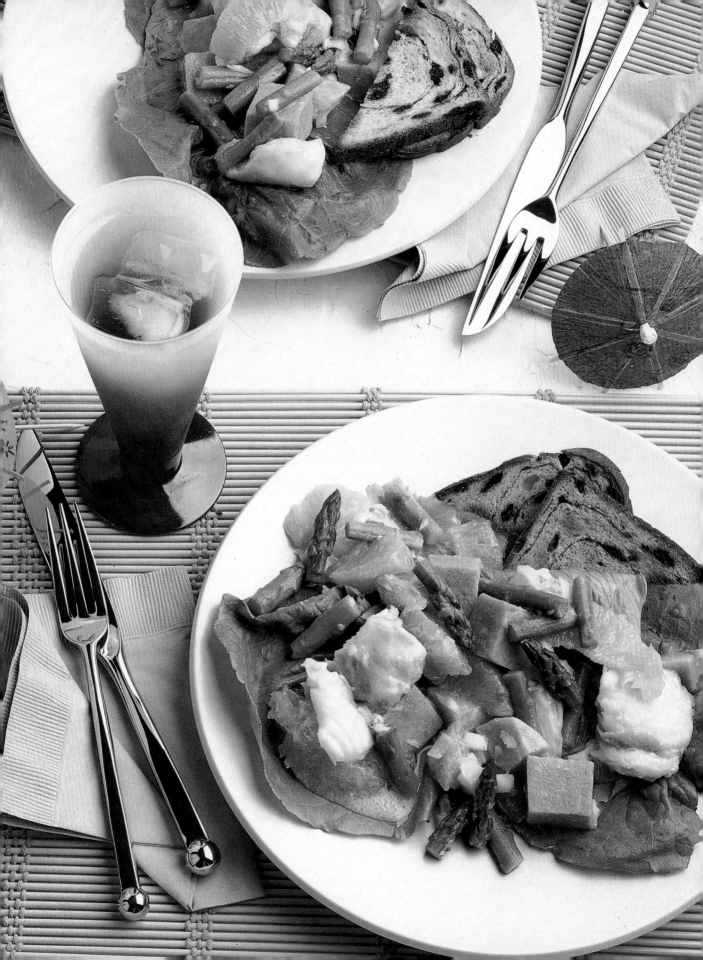

CALORIES per serving	331
62% Carbohydrate	52 g
24% Protein	21 g
14% Fat	5 g
CALCIUM	130 mg
IRON	5 mg
SODIUM	727 mg

SHRIMP MADRAS SANDWICH

Most shellfish is low in calories and cholesterol and rich in fluorine, a mineral that may help guard against calcium loss and osteoporosis.

2/3 cup yellow lentils
1 cup chopped onion
1 bay leaf
1 3/4 cups low-sodium stewed tomatoes with their liquid
1/2 cup chopped green bell pepper
1 tablespoon olive oil
1 tablespoon minced garlic
1 tablespoon minced fresh ginger
1 1/2 teaspoons ground coriander

1 teaspoon ground turmeric
3/4 teaspoon chili powder
1/4 pound shelled, deveined shrimp, cut in thirds
3/4 cup frozen green peas
3/4 teaspoon salt
1/8 teaspoon hot pepper sauce, or to taste
Four 2-ounce pita breads
1/4 cup plain lowfat yogurt

Place the lentils in a medium-size saucepan with 1 1/2 cups of water, the onion and bay leaf, and bring to a boil over medium-high heat. Cover the pan, reduce the heat to low and simmer for 30 minutes. Add the tomatoes and bell pepper, and cook for another 30 minutes, or until the lentils are tender. (The lentils can be cooked up to 2 days in advance and stored in the refrigerator.)

Heat the oil in a medium-size skillet over medium heat. Add the garlic and ginger and sauté for 1 minute. Add the coriander, turmeric and chili powder, and cook for another minute. Reduce the heat to medium-low, add the lentil mixture and cook for 5 minutes, or until thick. Add the shrimp, peas, salt and hot pepper sauce, and cook for 5 minutes, or until the shrimp are opaque.

Cut the pita breads in half crosswise (warm them slightly if desired) and fill each half with about 1/2 cup of the lentil mixture. Spoon 1 1/2 teaspoons of yogurt into each pita pocket and serve. Makes 4 servings

RASPBERRY FREEZE WITH LEMON SAUCE

Dieters need not give up dessert if they choose wisely. Instead of ice cream, made with egg yolks and heavy cream, have this freeze made with egg whites and lowfat milk. The dessert is also a good source of vitamin C.

Two 12-ounce packages frozen unsweetened raspberries (3 cups), partially thawed
1/2 cup frozen apple juice concentrate, thawed
1/2 cup lowfat milk (2%)
1/4 cup evaporated skimmed milk

1 1/2 teaspoons cornstarch
2 teaspoons grated lemon peel
2 large egg whites
2 tablespoons sugar
1 tablespoon lemon juice
2 tablespoons chopped fresh mint, plus mint sprigs for garnish

For the raspberry freeze, place the raspberries and apple juice concentrate in a food processor or blender and process until puréed. Put the purée through a food mill or force it through a sieve to remove the seeds, then transfer it to a freezer container and freeze it for at least 1 hour.

Meanwhile, make the sauce: In a medium-size saucepan stir together the lowfat milk, evaporated milk and cornstarch until smooth. Add 1 teaspoon of lemon peel and bring the mixture to a boil over medium heat, stirring constant-

CALORIES per serving	207
83% Carbohydrate	45 g
10% Protein	6 g
7% Fat	2 g
CALCIUM	132 mg
IRON	1 mg
SODIUM	68 mg

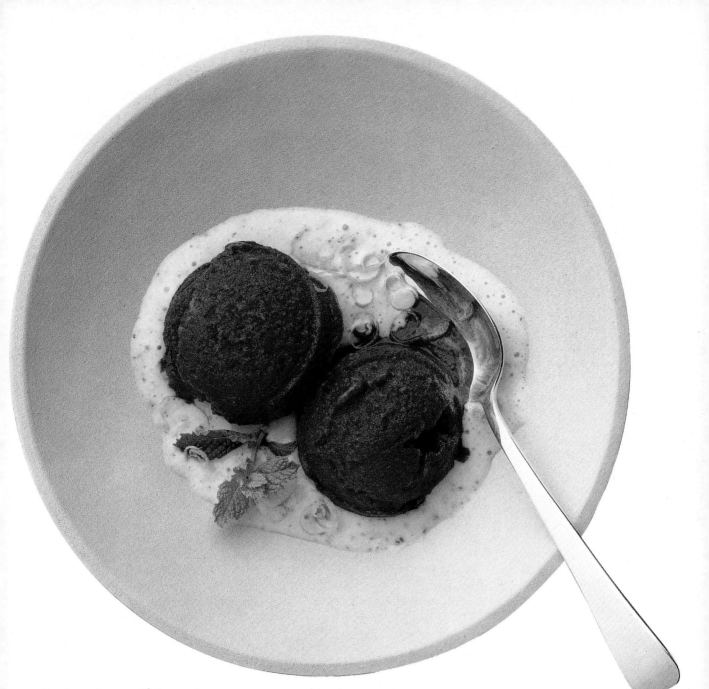

Raspberry Freeze with Lemon Sauce

ly; remove the pan from the heat and set aside. In a medium-size bowl whisk together the egg whites, sugar and lemon juice until frothy, then gradually whisk in the hot milk mixture. Return the mixture to the saucepan, add the mint and cook over low heat, stirring constantly, for 5 minutes, or until the sauce is thickened. Transfer the sauce to a small bowl, cover and refrigerate until well chilled.

To serve, let the raspberry mixture thaw at room temperature for 30 minutes, or until soft enough to scoop. Pour one fourth of the lemon sauce into each of 4 dessert dishes. Divide the raspberry freeze among the dishes and garnish with mint sprigs and the remaining lemon peel.   Makes 4 servings

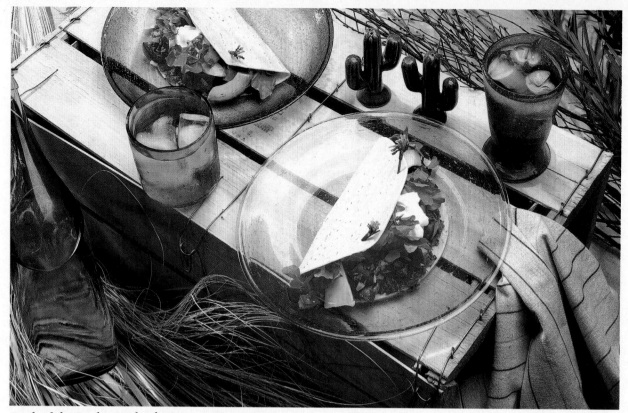

South of the Border Sandwiches

SOUTH OF THE BORDER SANDWICHES ▼

Beans, loaded with filling fiber, are usually cooked in lard and topped with sour cream in Mexican dishes. This recipe cuts the fat but not the flavor.

1/2 cup dried black beans
1 large tomato, coarsely chopped
1/4 cup chopped onion
1 tablespoon chopped
   fresh coriander
2 teaspoons balsamic vinegar,
   or to taste

4 medium-size flour tortillas
1/2 medium-size avocado
1/8 teaspoon salt
Pepper
3/4 cup watercress, washed
   and trimmed
1/4 cup plain lowfat yogurt

Place the beans in a medium-size saucepan with cold water to cover. Cover the pan and refrigerate the beans overnight.

Drain the beans, add 5 cups of fresh water and bring to a boil over medium-high heat. Reduce the heat to medium-low and simmer for 1 hour, or until the beans are soft. Drain, reserving 1 tablespoon of liquid; set aside to cool.

Preheat the oven to 350° F. For the salsa, in a small bowl stir together the tomato, onion, coriander and vinegar; set aside. Wrap the tortillas in foil and heat them in the oven for 5 minutes. Meanwhile, peel the avocado half and cut it into thin slices. Using a fork or potato masher, coarsely mash the beans, adding some of the cooking liquid if they are very dry. Stir in the salt and add pepper to taste.

Place each tortilla on a plate. Spread one half of each tortilla with one fourth of the beans, then divide the salsa, avocado slices, watercress and yogurt among them. Fold the tortillas over the filling and serve. Makes 4 servings

CALORIES per serving	241
61% Carbohydrate	38 g
16% Protein	10 g
23% Fat	6 g
CALCIUM	123 mg
IRON	4 mg
SODIUM	94 mg

ROASTED RED PEPPER SOUP WITH CROUTONS ▼

Soup is filling but usually low in calories because of its high water content. One study showed that dieters who had lowfat soups at least four times a week lost more weight than those who had soup less often.

4 large red bell peppers	1/4 teaspoon salt
1 small potato, boiled, peeled and quartered	1/4 teaspoon pepper
1 cup grated carrots	Three 1/2-inch-thick slices French bread (1 ounce total weight)
1 cup low-sodium chicken stock	1 tablespoon olive oil
1 cup lowfat milk (2%)	2 garlic cloves, minced

Preheat the broiler. Pierce the bell peppers in several places with a fork, place them on a broiler pan and broil them 6 inches from the heat, turning frequently, for 20 minutes, or until well charred. Place the peppers in a paper bag and let them steam for 15 minutes. Peel, seed and quarter the peppers and place them in a food processor with the potato, half the carrots, the stock, milk, salt and pepper. Purée the mixture until smooth, then transfer it to a medium-size saucepan and set aside.

Cut the bread into 1/2-inch cubes, place them a nonstick skillet with the oil and garlic and sauté over medium-high heat for 5 minutes, or until the croutons are crisp. Remove the pan from the heat. Heat the soup over medium heat for 5 minutes, ladle it into 4 bowls and garnish with the croutons and the remaining carrots.   Makes 4 servings

CALORIES per serving	142
56% Carbohydrate	21 g
12% Protein	5 g
32% Fat	5 g
CALCIUM	99 mg
IRON	2 mg
SODIUM	360 mg

TROPICAL BEAN SALAD

Adding a small amount of turkey (a complete protein) to this salad allows the body to make better use of the incomplete vegetable protein in the beans.

1/4 cup low-sodium chicken stock	3 1/2 cups cooked baby lima beans (2 cups dried)
2 tablespoons Dijon-style mustard	3 cups fresh pineapple chunks
2 tablespoons lemon juice	1 medium-size red onion, thinly sliced
4 teaspoons olive oil	
1 garlic clove, minced	6 plum tomatoes, cut into wedges
Black pepper	2 cups seedless grapes
3 tablespoons finely chopped fresh basil	2 ounces smoked turkey
1 large head Romaine lettuce	12 whole toasted almonds

For the dressing, in a small bowl combine the stock, mustard, lemon juice, oil and garlic. Add pepper to taste and whisk until smooth. Stir in the basil; set aside. Wash and trim the Romaine and cut the leaves in half crosswise; wrap the top halves in plastic wrap and refrigerate them. Cut the bottom halves of the leaves into very thin strips, place them in a large serving bowl, add the beans, pineapple, onion, tomatoes, grapes and turkey and toss gently to combine. Add the dressing and toss again. Cover the bowl and refrigerate for 3 hours, or until the salad is well chilled and the flavors blended.

To serve, arrange the reserved Romaine leaves around the edges of the salad. Scatter the almonds over the salad and serve.   Makes 6 servings

CALORIES per serving	378
63% Carbohydrate	63 g
18% Protein	18 g
19% Fat	8 g
CALCIUM	112 mg
IRON	7 mg
SODIUM	257 mg

VEGETABLE, CHICKEN AND CHEESE MELT

If you replace a thick slice of cheese on a toasted sandwich with grated or shredded cheese, you can use much less. It melts faster, too.

CALORIES per serving	305
56% Carbohydrate	44 g
23% Protein	18 g
21% Fat	7 g
CALCIUM	168 mg
IRON	3 mg
SODIUM	464 mg

1 tablespoon olive oil
1 cup chopped onion
2 garlic cloves, minced
3 red bell peppers, seeded and coarsely diced
2 medium-size zucchini, sliced 1/4 inch thick
Black pepper

1/4 pound boned, skinned chicken breast, cut into 1/2-inch chunks
Four 2-ounce whole-wheat pita breads
1/2 cup shredded part skim-milk mozzarella (2 ounces)
3 cups washed, stemmed watercress

Heat 2 1/2 teaspoons of oil in a medium-size nonstick skillet over medium heat. Add the onion and garlic, and cook, stirring, for 4 minutes. Increase the heat to medium-high, add the bell pepper and zucchini, and cook, stirring, for 5 minutes. Add 1/2 cup of water and cook for 3 minutes more. Add pepper to taste and, using a slotted spoon, transfer the vegetables to a bowl to cool. Add the chicken to the skillet and cook, stirring, over medium heat for 5 minutes, or until cooked through. Transfer the chicken to a small bowl. Wipe the skillet with paper towels; set aside.

Split the pita breads and sprinkle the bottom halves with mozzarella. Divide the vegetable mixture, chicken and watercress among the sandwiches and cover with the top halves of the pita breads. Heat the remaining oil in the skillet over medium-high heat. Place one sandwich at a time in the skillet and heat it for 3 minutes, or until the cheese melts, then carefully turn and heat it for 2 minutes more.

Makes 4 servings

Vegetable, Chicken and Cheese Melt

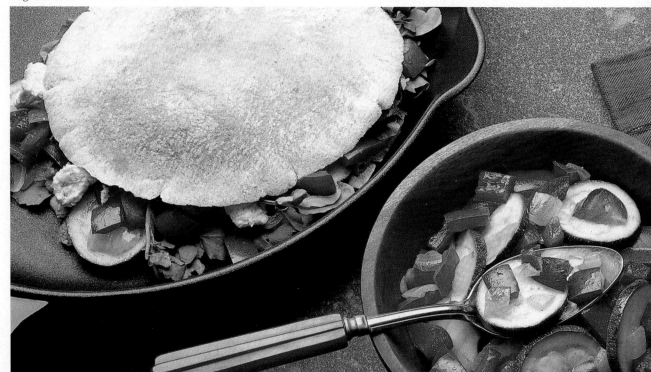

APPLE, FENNEL AND PASTA SALAD

This salad gives you more than 12 grams of dietary fiber, almost half the minimum daily fiber intake suggested by the American Dietetic Association.

CALORIES per serving	382
63% Carbohydrate	62 g
15% Protein	14 g
22% Fat	10 g
CALCIUM	241 mg
IRON	3 mg
SODIUM	576 mg

5 ounces elbow macaroni
1 1/2 cups frozen lima beans
1/4 cup balsamic vinegar
1 1/2 tablespoons olive oil
1 tablespoon frozen apple juice concentrate, thawed
2 teaspoons chopped fresh oregano, or 3/4 teaspoon dried oregano
1/2 teaspoon salt
1/4 teaspoon pepper
3 McIntosh apples (about 1 pound total weight)
2 tablespoons lemon juice
1/2 pound fennel bulb
2/3 cup thinly sliced radishes
1 1/2 ounces Parmesan
1/2 small head escarole

Bring a large saucepan of water to a boil. Add the macaroni and cook for 8 minutes, or according to the package directions until al dente; drain, rinse under cold water and set aside to drain thoroughly. Cook the lima beans according to the package directions; drain and set aside.

For the dressing, whisk together the vinegar, oil, apple juice concentrate, oregano, salt and pepper; set aside. Core but do not peel the apples, then dice them and toss them with the lemon juice in a large bowl. Trim and thinly slice the fennel and add it to the apples. Add the macaroni, lima beans, radishes and dressing, and toss well. Using a vegetable peeler or a sharp knife, cut the Parmesan into thin shavings; set aside.

To serve, wash and trim the escarole. Line a platter with escarole leaves and mound the apple mixture on top. Scatter the Parmesan shavings over the salad and serve.   Makes 4 servings

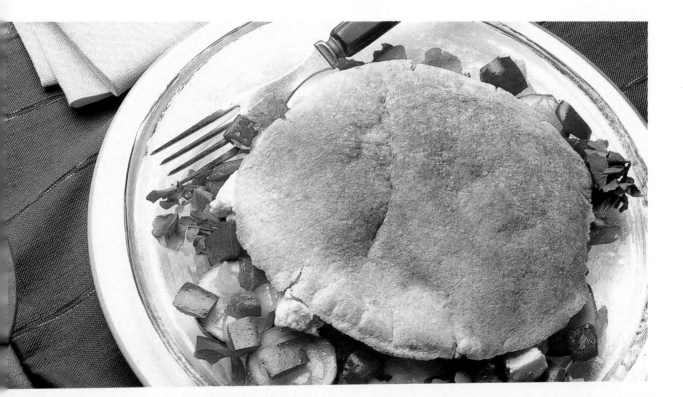

CALORIES per serving	141
65% Carbohydrate	24 g
15% Protein	6 g
20% Fat	3 g
CALCIUM	78 mg
IRON	1 mg
SODIUM	93 mg

LIME BAVARIAN

Using cream instead of skim milk here would add 550 calories.

1 1/2 teaspoons unflavored gelatin	2 large eggs, separated
1/4 cup freshly squeezed lime juice	4 tablespoons sugar
	Pinch of salt
3/4 cup skim milk	Pinch of cream of tartar
1 1/2 teaspoons grated lime peel	1 1/2 cups fresh blueberries

Sprinkle the gelatin over the lime juice in a cup and set aside to soften. Combine the milk and lime peel in a medium-size heavy-gauge saucepan and bring to a boil over medium heat. Remove from the heat and set aside to cool.

In a medium-size bowl, using an electric mixer, beat the egg yolks with 3 tablespoons of sugar until thick and pale. Whisk in the milk, return the mixture to the saucepan and cook over medium-low heat, stirring constantly, for 5 minutes, or until it coats the back of a spoon. Strain the mixture into the bowl, then add the gelatin mixture and stir until the gelatin is dissolved. Refrigerate, stirring occasionally, for 1 hour, or until the mixture begins to thicken.

In a large bowl, with clean beaters, beat the egg whites, salt and cream of tartar until foamy. Gradually beat in the remaining sugar and continue beating until soft peaks form. Fold the whites into the gelatin mixture. Spoon the Bavarian into 4 dessert dishes, cover and refrigerate for at least 4 hours. To serve, spoon some blueberries over each portion.   Makes 4 servings

Color can be a helpful guide to vitamin content when you choose fruits and vegetables. Generally, the deeper the color, the higher the nutrient content. For example, yellow corn (and cornmeal) has more vitamin A than white corn, and apricots have more than peaches. Oranges have more vitamin C and potassium than grapefruit. Acorn squash has more calcium and iron than crookneck squash, and kale is richer than lettuce in all nutrients.

SCALLOP AND ORANGE SALAD

Dark brown unhusked bulgur is one of the most nutritious forms of wheat.

2 navel oranges	2 tablespoons olive oil
1 1/3 cups orange juice	1/4 teaspoon each salt and pepper
6 ounces bay scallops	2 cups diced red bell pepper
2 tablespoons minced fresh ginger	2/3 cup thinly sliced scallions
1 tablespoon honey	1 cup raw bulgur
1 garlic clove, minced	3 cups leaf lettuce
1/4 cup white wine vinegar	2 cups broccoli florets, blanched

Grate 2 teaspoons of orange peel; set aside. Peel and section the oranges. Heat the orange juice in a large skillet over medium-high heat, add the scallops and cook for 30 seconds; drain in a strainer set over a bowl. Return the orange juice to the skillet, add the ginger, honey and garlic, and bring to a boil. Reduce the heat to low and cook, stirring occasionally, for 20 minutes, or until the liquid is reduced to 1/2 cup. Strain the liquid and set aside to cool.

In a large bowl whisk together the vinegar, oil, salt and pepper. Stir in the scallops, the orange liquid, orange sections, half the orange peel, the bell pepper and half the scallions; cover and refrigerate for 1 hour. Meanwhile, place the bulgur in a medium-size bowl and add 2 cups of cold water; set aside for 30 minutes, then thoroughly drain and squeeze it as dry as possible.

Line 4 plates with lettuce and divide the bulgur among them. Arrange the scallops, broccoli and oranges on top. Drizzle the dressing over the salads and sprinkle with the remaining scallions and orange peel.   Makes 4 servings

CALORIES per serving	391
65% Carbohydrate	67 g
16% Protein	16 g
19% Fat	9 g
CALCIUM	126 mg
IRON	5 mg
SODIUM	228 mg

Scallop and Orange Salad ▷

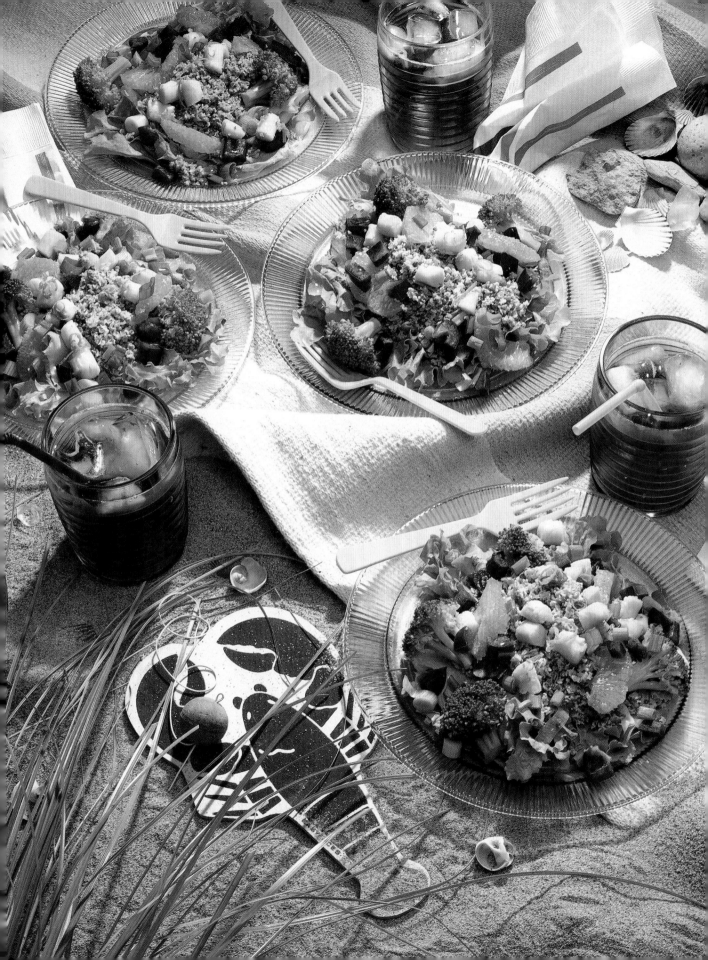

Mid-Afternoon Snacks

. . . .

EGGPLANT CAVIAR

Unlike most eggplant spreads, this one contains just a teaspoon of oil.

CALORIES per serving	144
69% Carbohydrate	27 g
14% Protein	6 g
17% Fat	3 g
CALCIUM	109 mg
IRON	2 mg
SODIUM	267 mg

2 1/4 pounds eggplant
1 red bell pepper
1 medium-size onion
1 garlic clove
1 tablespoon toasted
  sesame seeds

1 tablespoon chopped fresh parsley
1 teaspoon olive oil
1 teaspoon lemon juice
1/4 teaspoon salt
Black pepper
4 slices whole-wheat bread

Preheat the oven to 375° F. Prick the eggplant and bell pepper with a fork, place them on a baking sheet with the onion and bake for 45 minutes, or until the eggplant collapses and the onion is fork-tender; set aside to cool.

Halve the eggplant and scoop the flesh into a food processor or blender. Halve, stem and seed the pepper, and peel the onion and garlic. Add them to the eggplant. Process the mixture, pulsing the machine on and off, just until very coarsely chopped. Transfer the mixture to a bowl and stir in the sesame seeds, parsley, oil, lemon juice, salt, and pepper to taste. Cover and refrigerate the caviar for at least 1 hour. To serve, toast the bread, cut it into quarters and spread the caviar on it.   Makes 4 servings

Chewy Citrus Thins

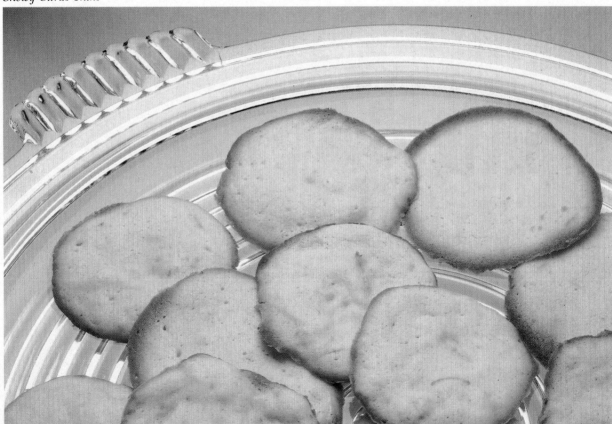

ZUCCHINI-RAISIN MUFFINS

Homemade whole-grain muffins make excellent snacks, but beware the oversized, oversweetened versions sold at snack counters: They often weigh as much as eight ounces and may have more than 650 calories.

CALORIES per muffin	149
60% Carbohydrate	24 g
13% Protein	5 g
27% Fat	5 g
CALCIUM	75 mg
IRON	2 mg
SODIUM	252 mg

Vegetable cooking spray
(optional)
1 cup rolled oats
1/2 cup ready-to-eat
whole-bran cereal
1 1/2 cups buttermilk
2 tablespoons margarine
2 tablespoons light brown sugar
1 large egg, lightly beaten

1 cup whole-wheat flour
1 teaspoon baking powder
1 teaspoon baking soda
1/4 teaspoon salt
1/4 teaspoon ground cinnamon
1 cup grated zucchini, squeezed dry
1/2 cup dark raisins
1/4 cup dry-roasted cashews,
coarsely chopped

Preheat the oven to 400° F. Spray 12 muffin-tin cups with cooking spray or line them with paper liners. In a medium-size bowl stir together the oats, cereal and buttermilk; set aside for 30 minutes.

In another medium-size bowl, using an electric mixer, cream together the margarine and brown sugar. Beat in the egg, then stir in the flour, baking powder, baking soda, salt and cinnamon. Add the flour mixture to the oats mixture and stir to combine. Stir in the zucchini, raisins and cashews, divide the batter among the muffin cups and bake for 35 minutes, or until a toothpick inserted in the center of a muffin comes out clean.   Makes 12 muffins

CHEWY CITRUS THINS

Pack a few of these almost fat-free cookies with a piece of fruit or a container of juice for an afternoon snack at work.

Vegetable cooking spray
4 teaspoons margarine, melted
and cooled
1 tablespoon lemon juice
2 teaspoons lime juice

1/3 cup unbleached all-purpose
flour
1/2 teaspoon grated lemon peel
1/4 teaspoon grated lime peel
1 large egg white
1/4 cup sugar

If the recommended intake of eight glasses of water a day seems excessive, you may be right. According to the Food and Nutrition Board of the National Academy of Sciences, your body requires one liter (a little more than a quart) of water for every 1,000 calories you consume. That means that if you are eating 1,500 calories per day, you need 1 1/2 quarts, or 6 eight-ounce glasses, daily. Remember, too, that you get a fair amount of water from certain foods, especially vegetables, fruits and soups, as well as from other beverages.

Preheat the oven to 350° F. Line two baking sheets with foil, spray with cooking spray and set aside. In a small bowl stir together the margarine and lemon and lime juice; set aside. In another small bowl combine the flour and lemon and lime peel. In a large bowl, using an electric mixer, beat the egg white until frothy. Gradually add the sugar, continuing to beat on high speed for about 3 minutes, or until glossy peaks form; set aside. Sprinkle the flour mixture over the egg white and gently fold it in, then sprinkle the margarine mixture over the batter and fold it in. Using a level tablespoonful of batter for each, form 6 cookies on each baking sheet, spreading the batter into a 3-inch circle with the back of the spoon. Bake for 10 to 15 minutes, or until the cookies are lightly browned around the edges. Let the cookies cool in the pan on a rack for 3 minutes, then peel them off the foil and place them on the rack to cool completely.   Makes 12 cookies

CALORIES per cookie	42
65% Carbohydrate	7 g
6% Protein	1 g
29% Fat	1 g
CALCIUM	2 mg
IRON	.1 mg
SODIUM	19 mg

FRUIT-BOWL DRINK

If your schedule includes after-work exercise, this lowfat, high-carbohydrate beverage is an ideal snack before or after your session.

1 1/4 cups orange juice		1/2 cup fresh pineapple chunks	
1 cup seeded watermelon chunks		1/4 cup unsweetened applesauce	
1/2 cup fresh raspberries		1 kiwi fruit, peeled	
1/2 cup fresh strawberries		1/2 medium-size pear	

Combine all of the ingredients in a food processor or blender and process until thick and smooth. Serve the drink over ice in 4 tall glasses.

Makes 4 servings

CALORIES per serving	101
89% Carbohydrate	24 g
5% Protein	1 g
6% Fat	1 g
CALCIUM	27 mg
IRON	1 mg
SODIUM	3 mg

SUNSET FRUIT MOLD

Packaged gelatin desserts have about 4 teaspoons of sugar per serving. Making your own fruit gelatin lets you control the sweetener, and a generous slice of this dessert gives you all the vitamin C you need daily.

Vegetable cooking spray	3 envelopes unflavored gelatin
1 cup fresh raspberries or frozen unsweetened raspberries	3/4 cup plain lowfat yogurt
	3 tablespoons honey
1 medium-size grapefruit	1 1/4 cups apricot nectar
1 medium-size orange	1 1/4 cups orange juice

Lightly spray a 6-cup ring mold with cooking spray. Arrange 8 raspberries in the bottom of the mold and set aside. Peel the grapefruit and orange, being careful to remove all the white pith. Working over a bowl to catch the juice, cut the fruit into sections; remove and discard the membranes. Cut the grapefruit sections in half; set aside the fruit and juice.

Place 3/4 cup of cold water in a small saucepan, sprinkle the gelatin over it and set aside for 5 minutes, then place over low heat and cook, stirring, for 5 minutes, or until the gelatin is completely dissolved. Combine the yogurt and 1 1/2 tablespoons of honey in a small bowl and stir in 2 tablespoons of the gelatin mixture; set aside.

In a large bowl combine the remaining gelatin mixture, the apricot nectar, orange juice and remaining honey. Set the bowl in another large bowl half filled with ice water and let stand, stirring occasionally, for 15 minutes, or until the mixture begins to thicken. Fold 3/4 cup of the fruit gelatin into the yogurt mixture and set aside.

Add the grapefruit and orange and their juice to the fruit gelatin and continue to chill it for about 20 minutes, or until it is thick enough to mound. Gently fold in the remaining raspberries and spoon the mixture into the prepared mold, leveling the surface with a spatula; refrigerate the mold. Place the bowl with the yogurt mixture in the bowl of ice water for 5 minutes, or until thickened, then spoon the yogurt mixture over the gelatin in the mold, spreading it evenly. Refrigerate the mold for 2 to 4 hours, or until firmly set.

To unmold the gelatin, run a knife around the edge to loosen it. Invert the mold on a large plate and shake it gently. If the gelatin does not release, place a towel wrung out in hot water over the inverted mold for about 1 minute, then gently shake the mold again.

Makes 8 servings

CALORIES per serving	112
81% Carbohydrate	24 g
14% Protein	4 g
5% Fat	1 g
CALCIUM	61 mg
IRON	.3 mg
SODIUM	19 mg

FRUIT FOLD-UPS

Pass up the 300-calorie pastries on the office snack cart, and treat yourself instead to one of these rich-tasting fruit- and nut-filled cookies.

1 cup unbleached all-purpose
   flour, approximately
2 tablespoons sugar
2 tablespoons margarine, well
   chilled
1/2 cup lowfat cottage cheese (1%)

1/2 cup dark raisins
3 tablespoons coarsely
   chopped walnuts
1/4 teaspoon ground cinnamon
1/4 teaspoon vanilla extract
3 tablespoons strawberry jam

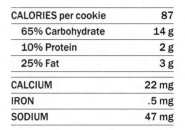

CALORIES per cookie	87
65% Carbohydrate	14 g
10% Protein	2 g
25% Fat	3 g
CALCIUM	22 mg
IRON	.5 mg
SODIUM	47 mg

In a medium-size bowl stir together 1 cup of flour and the sugar. Using a pastry blender or two knives, cut in the margarine until the mixture resembles coarse crumbs. Stir in the cottage cheese, gather the dough into a ball and knead it a few times in the bowl, then cover it loosely and refrigerate for 1 hour. Combine the raisins and walnuts on a cutting board and chop them finely; transfer to a small bowl and stir in the cinnamon and vanilla extract.

   Preheat the oven to 325° F. Line a large baking sheet with foil; set aside. Lightly flour the work surface and a rolling pin. Divide the dough into 2 equal pieces, roll out each piece into a 5 x 12-inch rectangle and place one rectangle with a long side toward you. Brush the bottom half with half of the jam, sprinkle it with half of the raisin mixture and fold the top half of the dough over to cover the filling. Cut the folded strip crosswise into eight 1 1/2-inch-wide cookies. Place the cookies 2 inches apart on the baking sheet and make 8 more cookies in the same fashion. Bake for 30 minutes, or until the cookies are golden brown, then transfer them to racks to cool.   Makes 16 cookies

Fruit Fold-ups

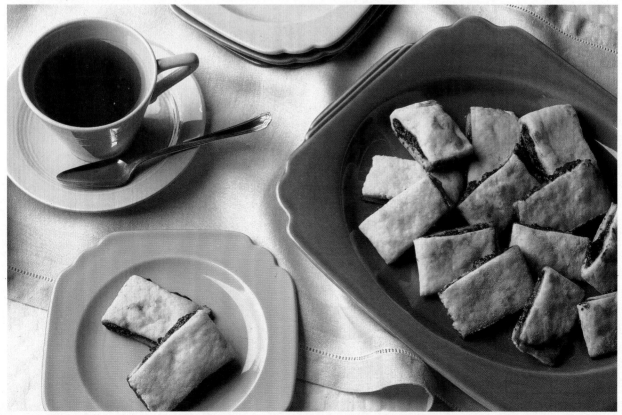

WHITE BEAN-CHEVRE SPREAD

Sour cream dips can turn low-calorie crudités into high-fat snacks. A bean purée flavored with herbs and a little cheese makes a healthier spread.

1 cup cooked, drained white beans
   (1/2 cup dried)
2 ounces chèvre (mild
   goat cheese)
1/2 cup chopped fresh parsley
2 tablespoons chopped fresh basil
2 tablespoons chopped
   fresh chives
1 tablespoon lemon juice
1/8 teaspoon salt

1/8 teaspoon pepper
12 asparagus stalks, trimmed
   and blanched
2 cups Brussels sprouts, blanched
4 small new potatoes, boiled and
   cut into large chunks
5 carrots, cut into sticks
2 each green and red bell peppers,
   cut into 1-inch-wide strips

CALORIES per serving	192
68% Carbohydrate	35 g
19% Protein	10 g
13% Fat	3 g
CALCIUM	86 mg
IRON	4 mg
SODIUM	184 mg

Place the beans, chèvre, herbs and lemon juice in a food processor or blender and process until puréed. Transfer the spread to a small serving bowl and stir in the salt and pepper. Arrange the vegetables in bowls and platters and serve with the spread.

Makes 6 servings

THREE-GRAIN BREADSTICKS

These peppery homemade breadsticks are satisfying between-meal snacks whether eaten alone or with a cup of soup or some lowfat cheese.

1 package active dry yeast
1 cup whole-wheat flour,
 approximately
1 cup unbleached all-purpose flour
1/2 cup rye flour

1 teaspoon coarsely ground pepper
1/2 teaspoon salt
Pinch of Cayenne pepper
Vegetable cooking spray
2 tablespoons cornmeal

Place the yeast in a large bowl, add 1 cup of warm water (105-115° F) and cover the bowl with plastic wrap; set aside for 10 minutes. In another large bowl combine 1 cup of whole-wheat flour, the all-purpose and rye flours, pepper, salt and Cayenne. Gradually stir the dry ingredients into the yeast mixture until a stiff dough forms. Turn the dough out onto a lightly floured work surface and knead it, adding more flour if necessary, for 8 to 10 minutes, or until the dough is smooth and elastic. Spray the bowl with cooking spray, place the dough in the bowl, cover with a kitchen towel and let rise in a warm place for 1 to 1 1/2 hours, or until the dough is doubled in bulk.

Preheat the oven to 350° F. Sprinkle two nonstick baking sheets lightly with cornmeal. Punch down the dough and knead it for 2 to 3 minutes, then let it rest for 10 minutes. Divide the dough into 4 equal pieces, then divide each piece into 10 equal parts. With floured hands, quickly roll each piece of dough into a stick about 12 inches long and 1/4 inch thick. Place the breadsticks on the baking sheets and bake for 15 to 20 minutes, or until lightly browned, switching the position of the baking sheets halfway through the baking time. Transfer the breadsticks to wire racks to cool, then leave at room temperature, uncovered, for 12 to 24 hours to crisp. Store the breadsticks loosely wrapped to keep them crisp. Makes 40 breadsticks

Because lean tissue — muscle — requires more fuel than fat does, your body uses 50 to 100 more calories per day for every pound of additional muscle you build: The more muscle you have, the more calories you burn, even at rest. Effective weight training will help you add lean muscle tissue.

CALORIES per breadstick	28
83% Carbohydrate	6 g
13% Protein	1 g
4% Fat	.1 g
CALCIUM	3 mg
IRON	.2 mg
SODIUM	28 mg

DRIED FRUIT PATTIES

Prunes and other dried fruits are excellent sources of minerals and fiber, and their concentrated natural sweetness helps satisfy a sugar craving.

1/2 teaspoon vegetable oil
20 dried apricot halves
10 dried apple slices

10 whole pitted prunes
12 whole unblanched almonds

Lightly oil the bowl and blade of a food processor. Cut 4 apricot halves into 16 thin strips; set aside. Place the remaining apricot halves, the apple slices, prunes and almonds in the processor and process until very finely chopped: The mixture should form a cohesive mass. Moisten your hands and shape the fruit mixture into a 6 x 1 1/2-inch log. Using a sharp knife dipped in hot water, cut the log into sixteen 1/4-inch-thick slices. If necessary, moisten your fingers again and reshape the slices into round patties. Place the patties on a baking sheet and press an apricot strip into the top of each one. Cover with plastic wrap and store the patties in the refrigerator. Makes 16 patties

Note: If you do not have a food processor, the ingredients can be chopped by hand. Lightly oil the knife blade to help keep the fruit from sticking to it.

CALORIES per patty	45
73% Carbohydrate	9 g
6% Protein	1 g
21% Fat	1 g
CALCIUM	10 mg
IRON	.4 mg
SODIUM	4 mg

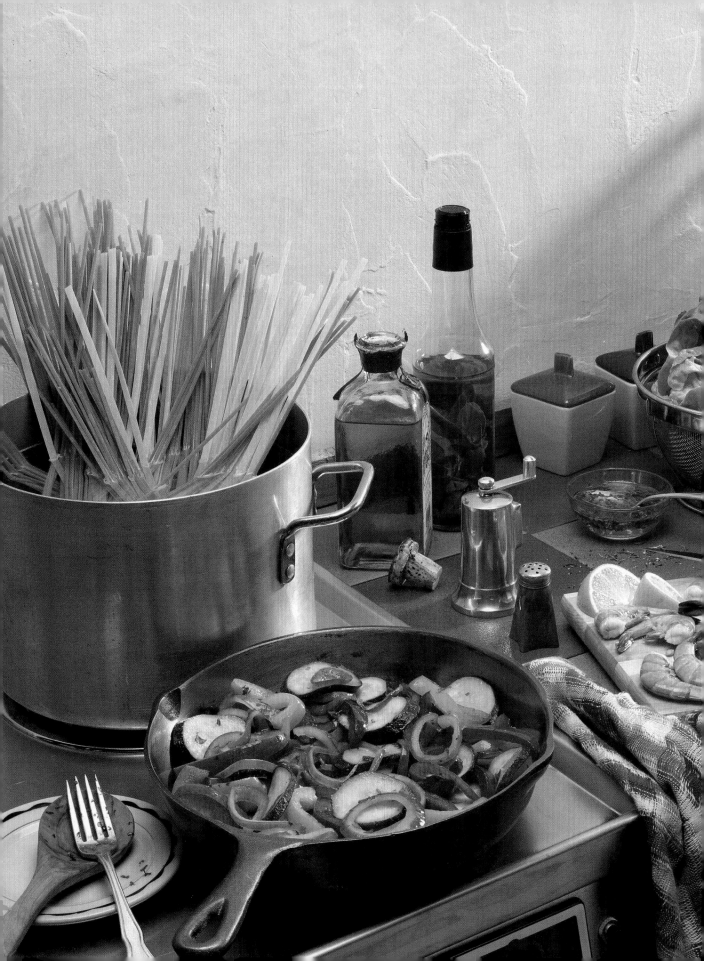

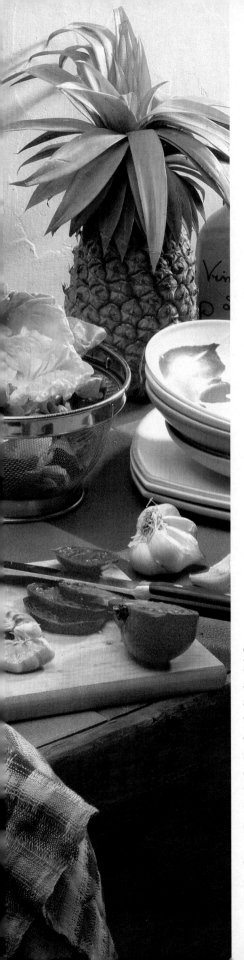

CHAPTER FOUR

Dinner

*Behavior-modification
strategies, alternatives to meat,
low-calorie desserts*

Limiting calorie intake at dinner is one of the most important elements of a successful weight-loss and -maintenance program. This meal, which can include an appetizer, main course, one or two side dishes, bread or rolls, beverage and dessert, usually constitutes the largest of the day. Although those on a weight-control plan sometimes skip breakfast or lunch, only rarely do they pass up dinner. Among the general population, a survey of food consumption patterns by the U.S. Department of Agriculture (USDA) found that Americans consume 42 to 45 percent of their total daily calories when they eat dinner. Most nutritionists recommend, however, that calorie consumption be more evenly distributed throughout the day.

The evening meal can be a difficult time for people who are cutting calories not only because of the amount of food offered to them, but also because of dinner's social aspect. The USDA survey found that almost 80 percent of American dinners are eaten with household

Most of the main-dish recipes in this chapter have from 300 to 399 calories per serving. Certain recipes, marked with a triangle, are extra-low in calories — between 170 and 275 per serving. Such recipes can be eaten as main dishes or combined with other foods. Three side dishes, all of which contain fewer than 150 calories, are also included. The desserts in this chapter have fewer than 275 calories.

members. And because this meal occurs at a time of day when you can put work-related pressures aside, dinner tends to be a more leisurely meal than breakfast or lunch — which may increase the temptation to overeat.

You can take steps to resist that temptation. In fact, the social aspect of dinner can actually aid you in eating smaller amounts. Put down your utensils between bites and make a point of talking to your companions. This will help you to avoid overly fast eating, a factor that has been linked with obesity. Another effective behavior-modification strategy is to condition yourself always to leave some food uneaten, which may be difficult at first if you were raised with the directive to finish everything on your plate.

You can also alter your eating environment when you eat at home. Remove the temptation for second helpings by having one person serve food from the kitchen, rather than serving family-style at the table. And switch from standard to smaller-size dinner plates to give the illusion of more food on each plate.

To satisfy your appetite with low-calorie food, begin dinner with a lowfat soup or a crunchy, fresh vegetable salad. Several studies have found that soup eaten before a meal will fill your stomach and so lead to lower total calorie consumption for the meal. Both this and the preceding chapter include several soups that are low in calories but rich in nutrients. Likewise, the fiber in raw vegetables such as red bell pepper and carrots — used in the Two-Rice and Pasta Salad on page 140 — will start to fill you up before you get to the main course.

Although the consumption of poultry has more than doubled in the United States in the past two decades, many dinners still center around servings of high-fat red meat that total eight ounces or more. Aside from the nutritional harm that the saturated fat in meat causes, particularly with regard to raising your cholesterol level, most red meat is very high in calories. An eight-ounce T-bone steak, for example, derives 60 percent of its 555 calories from fat. An eight-ounce chicken breast with the skin intact contributes 450 calories, of which nearly 40 percent are fat. Removing all visible fat from meat and the skin from poultry will significantly reduce their calorie and fat content. Far more effective than trimming fat from meat and poultry is to eat more lowfat fish and seafood, such as the Marinated Scallop Kebabs on page 118, instead. You can also substitute high-fiber grains for your entrees.

Many of the recipes that follow show you how to use meat as an adjunct to a meal, rather than as the centerpiece, with appetizing results that are low in calories. The Marinated Flank Steak with Pilaf on page 134, for example, uses only one and a quarter ounces of meat per portion, enough to give the dish a hearty flavor and some iron and B vitamins.

Besides containing a considerable portion of meat, many conventional dinner dishes are cooked in butter or oil, while others feature heavy cream sauces, marinades and stuffings — all of which add

Desserts

A considerable percentage of excess calories in the American diet comes from fat- and sugar-laden desserts. In fact, most Americans get nearly a quarter of their total daily calories from sugar. Giving up desserts is not necessary for a successful diet, but modifying your dessert choices may be. The following tips will help you lower your dessert calories:

◆ Choose fruit, either fresh or in combinations like compotes, in place of cakes, cookies and other baked goods, most of which are high in fat and heavily sweetened. You can make a fruit-yogurt parfait with alternating layers of the two ingredients. If you have canned fruit, check the label to see that it is canned in its own juice or in water, not sweetened syrup. To add variety to fruit desserts, stew or purée the fruit with cinnamon, nutmeg or other spices. Another possibility is to freeze fruits, such as grapes or bananas; eat them straight from the freezer, rather than thawing them, which makes their texture mushy.

◆ Decrease the sugar you use when you bake at home. In most recipes, sugar can be reduced by a third to a half without compromising the flavor of the dessert. Substituting brown sugar for white sugar does not cut calories — they are equal in calorie content, 16 calories per teaspoon, and equally devoid of vitamins and minerals. When you buy commercially prepared baked goods, read the labels. Fructose, dextrose, maltose, sucrose, corn syrup, sorbitol, xylitol and mannitol are all forms of sugar.

◆ Instead of a dish of ice cream or sherbet, finish your meal with a fruit-based sorbet. Sorbet contains approximately half the calories of premium ice cream and less than one percent fat. Other good choices are ice milk and lowfat frozen yogurt, with approximately 25 percent fewer calories than ice cream. Better still are frozen fruit bars: Those made with just fruit and fruit juice average only 70 calories a serving.

◆ If you have always thought of dessert as a reward for yourself, try to modify your behavior to focus on other nonfood pleasures. Get into the habit of taking a walk after dinner with family and friends, for example, or reading a magazine or a book.

unneeded fat. Cooking with a nonstick skillet and substituting wine, bouillon, lemon juice or soy sauce for oil or butter are important steps for preparing low-calorie dinner dishes. The trout recipe on page 130, for example, features a vegetable stuffing that does not depend on butter for flavor. Using lemon juice, yogurt and spices as salad dressings or as toppings for baked potatoes will also help you keep calories in check.

In addition to offering dessert recipes throughout this chapter that are low in calories, substitutions are suggested in the box above to enable you to include other desserts without paying the traditional toll in excess fat and sugar. Finally, one of the most difficult situations you may face while trying to lose weight is deciding what to eat when you are in a restaurant; the following two pages will guide you through menu choices and provide suggestions for eating at parties and other social occasions.

Dining Out

Many, if not most, people who embark on a weight-loss program find that dining out in restaurants can become their biggest challenge. As the chart on the opposite page indicates, a fair number of traditional menu entrees and side dishes are high in fat. And restaurants often increase the fat content of a dish by the way they prepare it — drenching a salad in oil, for example, or adding a mound of whipped cream to a piece of pie.

At the same time, there is a growing awareness among restaurant owners and food franchisers that the American public is interested in low-fat, low-calorie alternatives to traditional menu selections. In a recent study conducted by a public-opinion organization, more than half the 500 restaurant managers surveyed reported an increased demand for salads and seafood dishes. Three quarters of the respondents also said that they would alter their food-preparation methods if their customers asked them to do so.

The keys to dining out without overeating — be it at a restaurant, at a party or at a business gathering — are planning ahead and not allowing your motivation to falter. Here are some suggestions on how you can retain habits that help you control your weight when you eat away from home.

• Before you go out for a meal, have a low-calorie snack. Raw vegetables, a piece of fruit or a slice of lowfat cheese will help fill you up so that you are not tempted by the richer foods you may be offered at a restaurant or party.

• Pass up alcoholic drinks before, during and after dinner, or limit yourself to a glass of wine or beer. Exercising moderation has merit not only as a way to avoid unneeded calories: More than one drink tends to undermine your determination to restrain your eating. Of course, you can drink as much water before and during your meal as you want.

• Eat a few slices of bread before your dinner, preferably whole-grain bread, with a minimum of butter or margarine. Bread itself is low in fat and is relatively low in calories for its volume.

• Ask to have salad dressings served on the side. Avoid such toppings as olives, avocados and bacon, which are high in fat. If possible, make your own salad dressing of vinegar, oil and spices. Some of the most popular dressings served in restaurants are mayonnaise- or sour cream-based, and they get 90 percent of their calories from fat.

• Choose entrees and accompaniments chiefly from the center column on the opposite page. Use your judgment — and the recipes in this book — to identify other dishes that rank comparatively low in fat.

• Ask your waiter how certain foods are prepared. If the menu lists fried fish fillets, for example, you can ask that your fish be broiled with lemon juice instead of butter. You may be able to have such dishes as Salisbury steak and lobster Newburg served with a minimum amount of sauce, or with the sauce on the side. Some restaurants will cook chicken with the skin removed on request.

• Order fresh fruit for dessert. Fruit has more vitamins, minerals and fiber than ice cream, cake or pie, and fruit contains no fat.

WHAT TO ORDER

Choosing wisely from a menu is more than a matter of self-denial for those who are weight-conscious. If you prefer foods that get less than 30 percent of their calories from fat, select your meal from the middle column; the left-hand column contains items that are from 30 to 60 percent fat. The foods in the right-hand column are more than 60 percent fat.

OFTEN

Flounder

Chicken, white meat, no skin

Turkey, white meat no skin

Steamed crab

Lean ground sirloin

Veal, rump cut

Broiled shrimp

Steamed lobster

Spaghetti with tomato sauce

Fresh lean ham

Baked potato

Steamed vegetables

Green salad

OCCASIONALLY

Cod

Chicken, dark meat, no skin

Turkey, dark meat no skin

Smoked whitefish

Rib roast

Sirloin tips

Deviled crab

Lobster Newburg

Flank steak

Lean pork tenderloin

Mashed potatoes

French fries

Baked beans

RARELY

Mackerel

Fried chicken (including nuggets)

Duck

Deep-fried shrimp

Corned beef

Filet mignon

Leg of lamb

Fried crab

Salisbury steak with gravy

Pork spareribs

Olives

Coleslaw

Onion rings

Aerobic Workouts

Many studies have confirmed that aerobic exercise is the most efficient form of activity to burn off calories and thereby lose unwanted fat. For an exercise to be aerobic, it must provide continuous exertion for your body's major muscle groups. In order to cause the loss of body fat, the exercise must also be performed for a long enough time to expend a significant number of calories. Endurance activities, such as running, cross-country skiing, cycling, swimming and rowing, are aerobic exercises. Certain racquet sports can also produce a high calorie output if they are played intensely enough and at a sustained rhythm. The chart on the opposite page indicates the calorie values for different aerobic activities.

Based on guidelines established by the American College of Sports Medicine, you should exercise at least four days a week for 40 to 50 minutes, at a pace that raises your heart rate to within 60 to 75 percent of its maximum. If you are in good shape, you may do shorter, less frequent workouts at a slightly higher intensity: three days per week for 20 to 30 minutes per session, maintaining an intensity of at least 80 to 85 percent of your maximum heart rate. (These recommended times do not include your warm-up and cool-down.) Studies have shown that such a schedule is the minimum for any noticeable change in body composition or weight to occur.

To determine if you are exercising at the proper intensity, count your pulse for 10 seconds and multiply by six to obtain your heart rate. While you exercise, your heart rate should fall within a target zone that is 60 to 85 percent of its estimated maximum rate — which you can calculate by subtracting your age from 220. If you are 35 years old, for example, your target heart rate zone falls between 120 and 157 beats per minute.

During your workout, check your heart rate periodically to make sure you are exercising within your target heart rate zone. Once you have become accustomed to this level of intensity, you will begin to recognize when you have reached it without checking your pulse.

At each workout, you should warm up by performing your activity at an easy pace for five minutes, then build up the intensity. Exercise for at least 20 minutes within your target heart rate zone. Spend five minutes cooling down by gradually reducing the intensity of your workout.

The hardest part of an exercise program is doing it regularly. If running bores you, chances are that forcing yourself to complete a daily five-mile run will ultimately lead you to give it up. Instead, choose an exercise that you enjoy and that is accessible to you. The chart opposite lists some of the benefits that various exercises provide. You can also consider cross-training, or alternating two or more activities, such as bicycling and cross-country skiing.

An Exercise Guide

AEROBIC DANCE

This activity works all of your major muscles and can be performed either at home or in classes. If done at home, you can set your pace by your choice of music: Fast-tempo music will make the session more vigorous. Be sure your workouts are low-impact—one foot should be on the floor at all times—to reduce your chance of injury.

Light:	120
Moderate:	200
Vigorous:	300

CYCLING

A superb conditioner for the lower body, cycling can be performed outdoors or on an indoor stationary bike that allows you to adjust how hard you pedal. Outdoors, the injury rate is low, though cyclists should always wear hard-shell helmets for safety.

5.5 mph:	130
10 mph:	220
13 mph:	320

RACQUET SPORTS

Unlike the rhythmic movements of other aerobic activities, racquet sports alternate high- and low-intensity movements. Squash, racquetball and singles tennis are most effective for burning calories and for overall conditioning.

Badminton:	175
Tennis:	210
Racquetball:	360
Squash:	420

ROWING

Whether you row in a shell on the water or use an indoor machine, rowing is a powerful aerobic conditioner. It burns calories at a high rate, has a low injury rate and strengthens the whole body, particularly the thighs and upper back.

Light:	200
Vigorous:	420

RUNNING

A highly efficient exercise, running is also convenient and inexpensive. Competitive long-distance runners have less body fat than any other group of athletes. Running puts stress on the knees, lower legs and feet, so be sure to wear good running shoes that fit correctly.

5.5 mph:	320
6 mph:	350
7.5 mph:	430
10 mph:	550

SKIING

Both downhill and cross-country skiing can be excellent conditioners. Cross-country burns calories more effectively since you need not stop at the bottom of each hill. Cross-country skiing also strengthens the shoulders and upper arms.

Downhill:	300
Cross-country:	200-560

SWIMMING

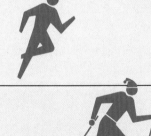

Many people, especially those who are overweight, find swimming an enjoyable exercise because it is free of weight-bearing stresses. The front crawl, or freestyle, is the most efficient stroke for an aerobic workout as well as being a good upper body conditioner.

25 yds/min:	180
40 yds/min:	260
50 yds/min:	375

WALKING

Certainly the most accessible exercise activity, walking is ideal if you are just starting an exercise program. You can increase the caloric expenditure of walking by increasing your pace and vigorously swinging your arms. Fast walking can burn more calories than running.

2.5 mph:	105
4.5 mph:	200
6 mph:	370

*Approximate caloric expenditure for a person weighing 150 lbs. Add 10 percent for every 15 lbs over this weight and subtract 10 percent for every 15 lbs under.

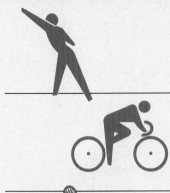

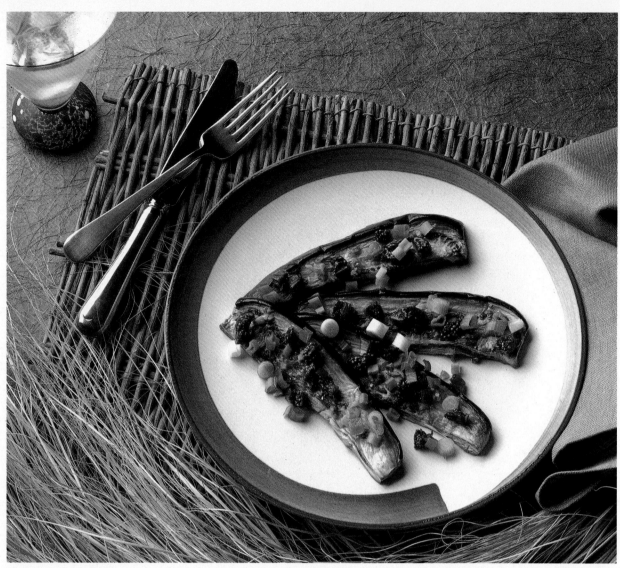

Chinese Baked Eggplant

CHINESE BAKED EGGPLANT ▼

A little chicken stock (instead of a lot of oil) keeps the eggplant moist during cooking. The small amount of dark toasted sesame oil in this recipe is used mainly for flavor.

1 1/2 pounds eggplant
1 tablespoon Oriental sesame oil
1 tablespoon minced fresh ginger
2 garlic cloves, chopped
Pinch of salt

Pepper
1/2 cup low-sodium chicken stock
2 dried Mission figs, chopped
 (2 ounces)
1/2 cup chopped scallions

CALORIES per serving	237
65% Carbohydrate	42 g
9% Protein	6 g
26% Fat	8 g
CALCIUM	186 mg
IRON	3 mg
SODIUM	96 mg

Preheat the oven to 375° F. Line a baking sheet with foil. Trim the eggplant and cut it in half lengthwise. Cut the halves lengthwise into 1/2-inch-thick slices, lay them on the baking sheet and sprinkle them with the oil, ginger, garlic, salt and pepper to taste. Drizzle the chicken stock over the eggplant, scatter the figs on top and bake for 30 minutes, or until the figs are golden brown. Top the eggplant with scallions and serve. Makes 2 servings

HERBED FETTUCCINE

If you find that a small portion of chicken or fish and a salad are not a filling meal, add a side dish of complex carbohydrates like this lightly sauced pasta.

3 garlic cloves

1 cup fresh basil leaves

2 tablespoons olive oil

1/2 cup low-sodium chicken stock

1/2 pound dried fettuccine

CALORIES per serving	149
60% Carbohydrate	22 g
11% Protein	4 g
29% Fat	5 g
CALCIUM	59 mg
IRON	2 mg
SODIUM	6 mg

Preheat the oven to 400° F. Place the unpeeled garlic cloves on a sheet of foil and bake them for 10 to 15 minutes, or until golden brown. Let the garlic cool slightly, then remove and discard the peel. Place the garlic cloves and basil in a food processor or blender and process for 15 to 30 seconds, or until finely chopped. With the machine running, slowly add the oil and stock; set aside.

Bring a large pot of water to a boil. Add the fettuccine and cook it for 10 to 12 minutes, or according to the package directions until al dente. Drain the fettuccine and transfer it to a serving bowl. Add the sauce and toss to combine. Serve immediately or, to serve the fettuccine chilled, refrigerate it for at least 3 hours.   Makes 8 servings

MOROCCAN STEW

Ethnic dishes add interest to a diet. Chickpeas are a good source of folacin, a vitamin necessary for red blood cell production.

1/2 pound acorn squash

1 medium-size zucchini

1 medium-size onion

2 carrots

1 cup low-sodium chicken stock

1/4 pound skinless, boneless
   chicken breast

One 14-ounce can plum tomatoes

1/2 cup cooked chickpeas

1/4 cup raisins or currants

2 teaspoons vegetable oil

1/4 teaspoon salt

1/8 teaspoon ground cinnamon

Dash of hot pepper sauce

1 cup instant couscous

2 tablespoons sliced
   toasted almonds

1 tablespoon chopped fresh mint

CALORIES per serving	388
66% Carbohydrate	59 g
21% Protein	19 g
13% Fat	5 g
CALCIUM	102 mg
IRON	3 mg
SODIUM	350 mg

Peel and seed the acorn squash and cut it into 1/2-inch dice. Trim the zucchini and cut it into 1/4-inch dice. Peel the onion and cut it into 1/4-inch dice. Peel and trim the carrots and cut them into 1/4-inch-thick diagonal slices.

Place the acorn squash, onion, carrots and stock in a medium-size saucepan, cover and cook over medium heat for 10 minutes, or until the vegetables are crisp-tender. Meanwhile, cut the chicken into 1-inch dice. Add the chicken, zucchini, the tomatoes and their liquid, the chickpeas, raisins, oil, salt, cinnamon and hot pepper sauce and cook, uncovered, over medium heat for 5 minutes, or until the vegetables are tender and the chicken is cooked through. Meanwhile, bring 1 cup of water to a boil in a small saucepan. Remove the pan from the heat, stir in the couscous, cover and let stand for 5 minutes.

To serve, fluff the couscous with a fork and mound it on a serving platter. Spoon the chicken mixture over the couscous and sprinkle it with the almonds and mint.   Makes 4 servings

MARINATED SCALLOP KEBABS ▼

This Mexican-style dish is a variation on seviche, which is made with uncooked seafood. This super-low-calorie meal supplies about one fourth of your protein requirement and all the vitamins A and C you need daily.

1/2 pound sea scallops, cleaned	2 tablespoons chopped
1/4 pound cherry tomatoes	fresh coriander
1/2 cup freshly squeezed	1 tablespoon grated orange peel
orange juice	1 large yellow or red bell pepper
3 tablespoons freshly	1 cup broccoli florets, blanched
squeezed lemon juice	Four 1-ounce rye rolls
1 tablespoon olive oil	

Bring 2 cups of water to a boil in a small saucepan. Add the scallops, reduce the heat to low and simmer for 1 to 2 minutes, or until the scallops are opaque and just firm; drain the scallops and place them in a medium-size nonreactive bowl. Add the tomatoes, orange juice, lemon juice, oil, coriander and orange peel, and stir to combine. Stem and seed the bell pepper, cut it into 1-inch squares and add it to the marinade. Add the broccoli, cover the bowl and place it in the refrigerator to marinate for 2 hours.

    To serve, thread the scallops, tomatoes, broccoli and bell pepper alternately on 8 long skewers and serve with the rolls.   Makes 4 servings

CALORIES per serving	195
52% Carbohydrate	26 g
28% Protein	14 g
20% Fat	5 g
CALCIUM	57 mg
IRON	3 mg
SODIUM	261 mg

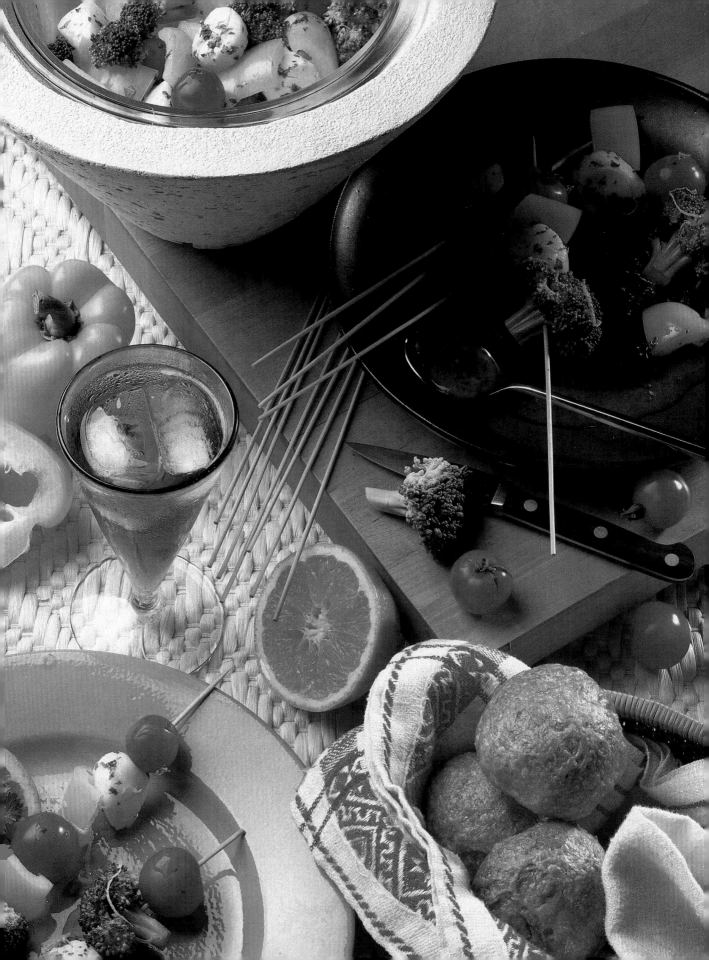

BEAN SOUP PAPRIKASH

If you sometimes overeat because you rush through your meals, have soup more often. A study showed that soup is eaten more slowly than other foods, thereby giving the brain more time to acknowledge that the stomach is full.

1 cup dried kidney beans	2 cups low-sodium stewed
2/3 cup dried pinto beans	tomatoes with their liquid
2 large onions, peeled	2 tablespoons paprika
2 large garlic cloves, peeled	1 teaspoon dry mustard
1 pound potatoes	2 1/2 tablespoons barley
2 large carrots	1/4 cup red wine vinegar
6 ounces green cabbage	Pepper
1 slice smoked bacon, diced	1/4 cup lowfat sour cream
4 cups low-sodium beef stock	

Place the beans in a medium-size saucepan, add 3 cups of water and bring to a simmer over medium heat. Cook for 2 minutes, then remove the pan from the heat, cover and let stand for 1 hour. Drain the beans, add 1 onion, 1 garlic clove and 2 cups of water, and bring to a boil over medium-high heat. Reduce the heat to low and simmer for 1 hour, or until the beans are almost tender. Meanwhile, chop the remaining onion and garlic. Scrub the potatoes and cut them into 1-inch cubes. Trim, peel and slice the carrots. Wash and trim the cabbage and cut it into 1-inch chunks; set aside.

Sauté the bacon in a large stockpot until browned. Add the chopped onion and garlic and cook for 5 minutes, or until soft. Add the stock, tomatoes, paprika and mustard and bring to a boil. Add the barley, potatoes and carrots and cook for 45 minutes.

Remove and discard the onion and garlic from the beans and add the beans and their liquid to the soup. Add the cabbage and cook for 15 minutes, or until the vegetables are tender. Stir in the vinegar and add pepper to taste. Ladle the soup into 4 bowls and garnish with sour cream.   Makes 6 servings

CALORIES per serving	382
71% Carbohydrate	71 g
18% Protein	18 g
11% Fat	5 g
CALCIUM	139 mg
IRON	6 mg
SODIUM	85 mg

F or cooking, use unhydrogenated oils *that are high in polyunsaturated or monounsaturated fats. Safflower, sunflower, corn, soybean, cottonseed and olive oils are good choices. But bear in mind that despite the nutritional advantage of nonsaturated fats, all oils are 100 percent fat and have the same calorie count — about 120 calories per tablespoon.*

BROWN RICE SAUTE ▼

The vegetables in this one-skillet meal provide more than 2,700 milligrams of vitamin A and, with the walnuts and brown rice, a good deal of fiber.

1 tablespoon corn oil	1 cup chopped scallions
1 garlic clove, chopped	Pinch of salt
2 1/2 cups cooked brown rice	1/4 teaspoon pepper
(about 3/4 cup raw)	1/2 ounce walnut halves (8 to 10)
1 cup sliced yellow squash	1 tablespoon grated orange peel
1 cup diced red bell pepper	1 tablespoon chopped fresh parsley

Heat the oil in a medium-size skillet over medium heat. Add the garlic, and sauté for 2 to 3 minutes. Add the rice, squash, bell pepper, scallions, salt, pepper and 1/4 cup of water and bring the mixture to a boil over high heat. Reduce the heat to medium-low and simmer, stirring constantly, for 5 minutes, or until the squash and peppers are tender. Stir in the walnuts, orange peel and parsley and serve.   Makes 4 servings

CALORIES per serving	219
65% Carbohydrate	36 g
8% Protein	5 g
27% Fat	7 g
CALCIUM	44 mg
IRON	2 mg
SODIUM	36 mg

GREEK SALAD ▼

Eliminating the oil and olives from a Greek salad cuts fat and calories considerably; a yogurt dressing and black-eyed peas are used instead.

1 large cucumber
1/2 cup plain lowfat yogurt
1/4 cup chopped fresh mint
3 tablespoons lemon juice
1 teaspoon sugar
4 plum tomatoes

1/4 pound Romaine lettuce, torn
  into bite-size pieces
2 cups cooked black-eyed peas
  (1 cup dried)
1/4 cup chopped scallions
1 ounce feta cheese, crumbled

CALORIES per serving	170
63% Carbohydrate	28 g
24% Protein	11 g
13% Fat	3 g
CALCIUM	142 mg
IRON	3 mg
SODIUM	123 mg

For the dressing, scrub the cucumber and halve it lengthwise. Peel and seed one half, cut it into large chunks and process it in a food processor or blender for 15 to 20 seconds, or until puréed. Add the yogurt, mint, lemon juice and sugar and process for another 5 to 10 seconds, scraping down the sides of the container with a rubber spatula; set aside. Cut the remaining cucumber half lengthwise into quarters, then cut it crosswise into 1/4-inch-thick slices. Cut the tomatoes into large dice. Place the Romaine, cucumber, tomatoes, peas and scallions in a large bowl and toss to combine. Sprinkle the feta over the salad and, just before serving, add the dressing and toss the salad.

Makes 4 servings

Greek Salad

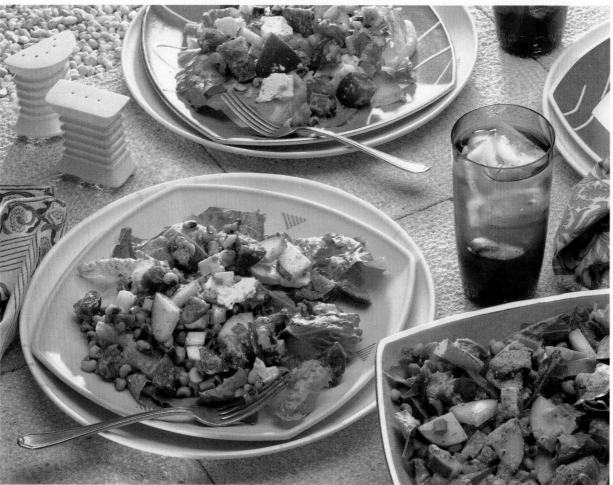

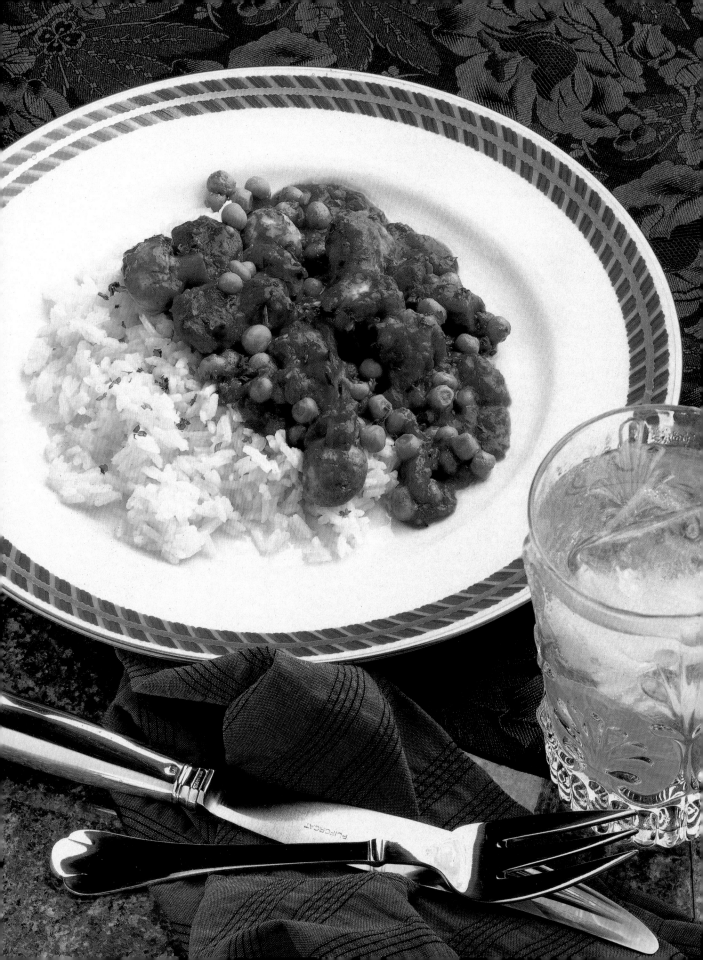

LAMB AND MUSHROOM STEW WITH ROSEMARY

Lowfat diets often lack niacin, which helps the body use energy from foods. This stew supplies more than half of a woman's daily niacin quota.

2 tablespoons unbleached
  all-purpose flour
1/4 teaspoon each salt and pepper
1/2 pound lean stewing lamb, cut
  into 1-inch cubes
1 tablespoon vegetable oil
One 14-ounce can plum tomatoes
1/4 pound small fresh mushrooms
1 garlic clove, crushed and peeled

1 bay leaf
3/4 teaspoon fresh rosemary, or
  1/4 teaspoon dried rosemary,
  chopped
2 tablespoons chopped fresh
  parsley
1 cup long-grain white rice
1/2 cup frozen peas, thawed

CALORIES per serving	352
59% Carbohydrate	51 g
19% Protein	17 g
22% Fat	8 g
CALCIUM	61 mg
IRON	4 mg
SODIUM	339 mg

Mix the flour, salt and pepper on a sheet of waxed paper and dredge the lamb cubes in the mixture. Reserve the excess flour. Heat the oil in a medium-size saucepan over medium heat, add the lamb and sauté for 5 to 10 minutes, or until the meat is well browned all over.

Add the remaining flour mixture and cook, stirring, for 1 minute. Add the tomatoes and their liquid, the mushrooms, garlic, bay leaf, rosemary and 1 tablespoon of parsley and bring to a boil. Reduce the heat to medium-low, cover the pan and simmer the stew for 30 minutes. Meanwhile, bring 3 cups of water to a boil in a medium-size saucepan. Stir in the rice, cover the pan, reduce the heat to medium-low and simmer for 20 minutes, or until the rice is tender and the water is completely absorbed. Remove the bay leaf from the stew and stir in the peas. Divide the rice among 4 plates, spoon the stew over it and sprinkle with the remaining parsley.   Makes 4 servings

If you love cheese, it is hard to give it up for a lowfat diet; however, if you select cheese carefully and limit the amount you eat, you can still cut fat and calories. Almost all hard cheeses are high in fat, but if you choose sharp, flavorful ones like sharp Cheddar or Parmesan, just a sprinkling is enough. Even part skim-milk mozzarella is about 60 percent fat, but when finely shredded, a little will suffice.

CAULIFLOWER-CHEESE SOUP

A bowlful of this thick puréed soup supplies your full daily requirement of vitamin C, most of it from the sweet potato and cauliflower.

1 tablespoon butter
1 cup chopped leeks
2 cups low-sodium chicken stock
One large sweet potato
  (about 14 ounces), peeled and
  cut into 1/2-inch-thick slices

4 cups cauliflower florets
1 tablespoon coarse-grain mustard
2 tablespoons chopped
  fresh parsley
1/3 cup grated Swiss cheese
4 small pita breads

Heat the butter in a medium-size saucepan over medium heat. Add the leeks, and sauté for 3 to 5 minutes, or until tender. Add the stock and 1 cup of water and bring to a boil. Add the potato and cauliflower, reduce the heat to low, cover the pan and simmer for about 20 minutes, or until the potato is tender.

Remove the pan from the heat and allow the soup to cool slightly. Transfer the soup to a food processor or blender, in batches if necessary, and process it for 1 to 2 minutes, or until puréed, scraping down the sides of the container with a rubber spatula. Stir in the mustard and parsley, ladle the soup into 4 bowls and top each serving with grated cheese. Serve the pita breads, warmed if desired, with the soup.   Makes 4 servings

CALORIES per serving	320
67% Carbohydrate	54 g
15% Protein	12 g
18% Fat	7 g
CALCIUM	166 mg
IRON	3 mg
SODIUM	418 mg

ITALIAN SPLIT-PEA STEW

CALORIES per serving	341
67% Carbohydrate	61 g
20% Protein	18 g
13% Fat	5 g
CALCIUM	133 mg
IRON	5 mg
SODIUM	604 mg

Without the traditional ham or sausage, split-pea stew becomes a lowfat dish; it is also an excellent source of B vitamins, potassium and fiber.

1 tablespoon butter	1 cup dried yellow split peas
1 1/2 cups chopped onions	3/4 teaspoon dried oregano
1 garlic clove, chopped	1 bay leaf
One 35-ounce can plum tomatoes	4 whole wheat rolls (2 ounces each)

Heat the butter in a medium-size saucepan over medium heat. Add the onions and garlic and sauté for 10 minutes, or until golden. Add the tomatoes and their liquid, the split peas, oregano, bay leaf and 1 cup of water and bring to a boil. Reduce the heat to medium-low, cover the pan and simmer the stew for 25 minutes, or until the peas are tender. Ten minutes before serving, warm the rolls in a 350° F oven or toaster oven.

To serve, remove and discard the bay leaf, ladle the stew into 4 bowls and serve with the warm rolls. Makes 4 servings

LENTILS WITH GOAT CHEESE DRESSING

CALORIES per serving	293
53% Carbohydrate	40 g
17% Protein	13 g
30% Fat	10 g
CALCIUM	121 mg
IRON	5 mg
SODIUM	386 mg

Although more popular as a soup ingredient, lentils are also a good basis for a dinner salad. Combining the lentils, which are legumes, with a grain such as brown rice gives you complete protein: The amino acids lacking in the lentils are supplied by the rice. Adding cheese and chicken stock, which are complete proteins, further enhances your protein intake from this meal.

1 cup dried lentils	2 teaspoons Dijon mustard
2 cups diced red onions	2 ounces mild goat cheese, such as
1/2 cup finely chopped scallions	Montrachet
1 cup grated carrots	1/2 teaspoon salt
1 cup cooked brown rice	Pepper
(1/3 cup raw)	4 cups thinly sliced red cabbage
1 teaspoon grated lemon peel	(1/2 pound)
1/2 cup low-sodium chicken stock	4 cups shredded spinach
1/4 cup red wine vinegar,	1 cup slivered red bell pepper
preferably balsamic	3/4 cup julienned radishes
3 tablespoons vegetable oil	1/2 cup finely chopped fresh parsley

Place the lentils and 3 cups of water in a medium-size saucepan and bring to a boil over medium heat. Reduce the heat to low and simmer for about 25 minutes, or until the lentils are soft. Drain any liquid and transfer the lentils to a medium-size bowl to cool. Add the onions, scallions, carrots, rice and lemon peel and toss to combine; set aside.

For the dressing, process the stock, vinegar, oil, mustard, cheese, salt, and pepper to taste in a food processor or blender until well blended. Pour the dressing over the lentil mixture and stir to combine; set aside for about 30 minutes to allow the flavors to blend.

To serve, make a bed of cabbage and spinach on a large serving platter and mound the lentil salad on top. Garnish with the bell pepper, radishes and parsley and serve. Makes 6 servings

TRUE GRIT VANILLA PUDDING

If you enjoy ice cream for dessert, try this pudding instead. It has a creamy, rich texture with just a fraction of ice cream's fat and sugar.

CALORIES per serving	233
55% Carbohydrate	32 g
18% Protein	10 g
27% Fat	7 g
CALCIUM	253 mg
IRON	1 mg
SODIUM	111 mg

1 cup skim milk

1/4 cup quick-cooking grits

1/4 cup sugar

2 teaspoons unsalted butter

1/2 teaspoon vanilla extract

1 cup part skim-milk ricotta cheese

2 kiwi fruits

Bring the milk to a boil in a small saucepan over medium heat and slowly stir in the grits. Return the milk to a boil, reduce the heat to low and cook, stirring occasionally, for 3 to 4 minutes, or until the mixture is as thick as cooked oatmeal. Remove the pan from the heat, add the sugar, butter and vanilla and stir until smooth; set aside to cool for about 5 minutes.

Process the ricotta in a food processor or blender until smooth. Add the cooled grits and process until smooth. Divide the pudding among 4 dessert dishes and refrigerate for at least 1 hour.

Just before serving, peel the kiwi fruits and cut them into 1/4-inch-thick slices. Arrange a few slices on top of each pudding.   Makes 4 servings

True Grit Vanilla Pudding

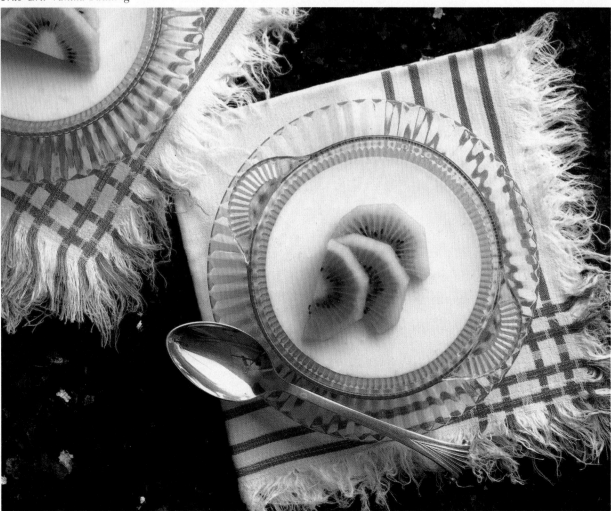

CABBAGE-CARROT-BEAN SOUP

CALORIES per serving	360
80% Carbohydrate	50 g
17% Protein	16 g
3% Fat	1 g
CALCIUM	190 mg
IRON	6 mg
SODIUM	188 mg

A serving of this soup has only 188 milligrams of sodium, compared with canned bean or vegetable soup, which may have 800 milligrams per cup.

1 cup dried pinto beans
1 1/2 cups chopped onions
2 garlic cloves, chopped
1/4 cup chopped fresh dill
1 bay leaf
1/4 teaspoon salt
1/4 teaspoon pepper

3 1/2 cups peeled, diced sweet potatoes
4 cups thickly sliced green cabbage
1 cup sliced carrots
1 cup sliced yellow squash
1/4 cup chopped fresh parsley

Place the beans in a large pot, add enough cold water to cover them and refrigerate them overnight.

Rinse and drain the beans and return them to the pot. Stir in the onions, garlic, 3 tablespoons of dill, the bay leaf, salt and pepper. Add the potatoes and 2 quarts of water and bring to a boil over medium-high heat. Reduce the heat to medium-low, cover the pot and simmer for 35 to 45 minutes, or until the beans are tender.

Add the cabbage, carrots and squash and return the soup to a boil. Cook for another 5 to 10 minutes, or until the carrots are tender. Remove and discard the bay leaf, then stir in the parsley. Ladle the soup into 4 bowls and garnish with the remaining dill. Makes 4 servings

L abels can be source of confusion when you shop for reduced-calorie foods. "Sugarless" foods may contain glucose or fructose, both sugars. "Light" foods may be light in color, texture or flavor — but not in calories or fat. "Natural" can mean just about anything. Check the nutrition chart on the package, then read the ingredients carefully and learn to recognize the hidden sugars, fats and additives you wish to avoid.

Cabbage-Carrot-Bean Soup

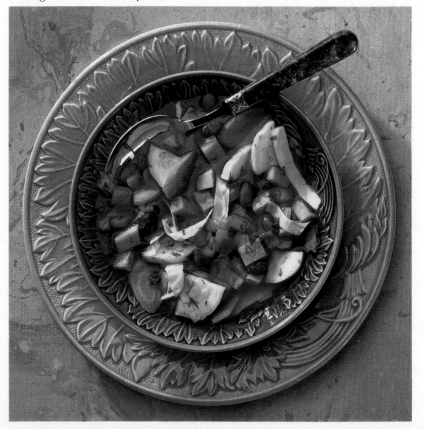

POTATO-VEGETABLE SALAD WITH SALMON ▼

Leaving out the mayonnaise and adding fish and an abundance of low-calorie vegetables turns potato salad into a lowfat dinner dish. Adding salt at the last minute means that you taste it more, so you can use less.

CALORIES per serving	213
54% Carbohydrate	30 g
17% Protein	9 g
29% Fat	7 g
CALCIUM	122 mg
IRON	2 mg
SODIUM	275 mg

1/2 cup plain lowfat yogurt
2 tablespoons plus 1 teaspoon
  olive oil
2 tablespoons finely chopped
  fresh dill
1 tablespoon Dijon-style mustard
1/4 teaspoon pepper
1 1/2 pounds small red potatoes,
  boiled, peeled and quartered
1/2 pound green beans, cut into
  1-inch lengths and blanched

1 1/3 cups grated zucchini
1 cup grated carrots
1 cup finely shredded red cabbage
3/4 cup thinly sliced radishes
1/2 cup frozen lima beans, blanched
One 3 3/4-ounce can water-packed
  salmon
2 shallots, finely chopped
1 tablespoon chopped fresh parsley
1/4 teaspoon salt

For the dressing, in a small bowl stir together the yogurt, oil, dill, mustard and pepper until well blended; set aside. Place the potatoes, green beans, zucchini, carrots, cabbage, radishes and lima beans in a large bowl and stir to combine. Drain the salmon and add it to the salad. Add the shallots, parsley and dressing and stir gently, breaking up the salmon as little as possible. Add the salt, stir again and serve.   Makes 6 servings

PEAR BREAD PUDDING

When you leave out the butter and use skim milk, bread pudding is a lowfat, high-carbohydrate dessert. The fiber in the whole-wheat bread and pears not only makes you feel full, but also helps lower blood cholesterol levels.

CALORIES per serving	228
70% Carbohydrate	41 g
14% Protein	8 g
16% Fat	4 g
CALCIUM	126 mg
IRON	2 mg
SODIUM	188 mg

2 large eggs
2 tablespoons unbleached
  all-purpose flour
2 tablespoons sugar
1 cup skim milk
1 teaspoon grated lemon peel
1 teaspoon almond extract

4 slices whole-wheat bread,
  preferably slightly stale,
  cut into 1/2-inch cubes
2 ripe pears (18 ounces
  total weight), peeled, cored
  and cut into 1/2-inch cubes

Preheat the oven to 375° F. Break the eggs into a small bowl and lightly beat them; set aside. For the custard, in a medium-size bowl stir together the flour and sugar. Gradually add the milk, beating the mixture constantly to prevent lumps from forming. Stir in the eggs, lemon peel and almond extract. Combine the bread cubes and pears and divide them among four 8-ounce custard cups or ramekins. Pour the custard over the bread and pears (it will not completely cover them) and stir gently to coat. Bake the puddings for 25 to 30 minutes, or until the custard is set and golden brown on top. Serve the pudding hot, at room temperature or chilled.   Makes 4 servings

FARINA POLENTA WITH CHEESE ▼

Enriched hot breakfast cereal, an excellent source of iron, can be a dinner ingredient, too. A serving of this cheese-topped farina cake provides more than 9 milligrams of iron — as much as 9 ounces of roast beef.

3/4 cup coarsely chopped onion	1/4 teaspoon pepper
2 garlic cloves, finely chopped	1 tablespoon chopped fresh dill
2 teaspoons butter	2 teaspoons curry powder
1 cup diced zucchini	2/3 cup enriched farina
1 cup diced red bell pepper	2 tablespoons grated
1/4 teaspoon salt	Cheddar cheese

In a medium-size, heavy-gauge ovenproof skillet, sauté the onion and garlic in the butter over medium heat for 4 minutes, or until the garlic is golden. Add the zucchini and bell pepper and cook, stirring, for 1 to 2 minutes more, adding up to 2 tablespoons of water, if necessary, to prevent sticking. Add the salt, pepper, dill and curry powder, cover the pan, reduce the heat to low and cook for 5 to 7 minutes, or until the vegetables are tender.

Preheat the broiler. Bring 2 3/4 cups of water to a boil in a small saucepan over medium heat. Add the farina, whisking constantly for about 30 seconds to prevent lumps from forming. Pour the farina over the vegetables, stir gently to combine and sprinkle with cheese. Broil the polenta 6 inches from the heat for about 1 minute, or until the cheese is melted.   Makes 4 servings

CALORIES per serving	170
67% Carbohydrate	28 g
12% Protein	5 g
21% Fat	4 g
CALCIUM	94 mg
IRON	9 mg
SODIUM	182 mg

LENTIL MINESTRONE

Even though this soup contains very small amounts of meat and cheese, it provides 14 grams of protein in a 286-calorie serving. Much of the protein comes from the lentils and macaroni.

1 teaspoon olive oil	4 small green tomatoes,
2 ounces ground chuck	cut into 1-inch cubes
1 1/2 cups coarsely	2 ounces elbow macaroni
chopped onions	1 bay leaf
2 cups coarsely diced bell peppers	1 tablespoon lime juice
1 cup diced celery	3/4 teaspoon salt
2 garlic cloves, minced	1/2 teaspoon dried oregano
1/3 cup dried lentils	Black pepper
1/4 cup white rice	1/4 cup grated Parmesan

Heat the oil in a Dutch oven or large heavy-gauge saucepan over medium heat. Add the ground chuck, onions, bell peppers, celery and garlic and cook, stirring, for about 5 minutes, or until the vegetables are softened. Stir in the lentils, rice, tomatoes, macaroni, bay leaf and 2 quarts of water, cover the pan and bring to a boil. Reduce the heat to low and simmer for 45 minutes.

Add the lime juice, salt, oregano, and pepper to taste. Remove and discard the bay leaf, ladle the soup into 4 bowls and sprinkle it with Parmesan.

Makes 4 servings

CALORIES per serving	286
61% Carbohydrate	44 g
19% Protein	14 g
20% Fat	7 g
CALCIUM	142 mg
IRON	4 mg
SODIUM	563 mg

ORZO VEGETABLE SALAD

Orzo is a pasta shaped like rice. Enriched pasta is a good low-calorie source of the B vitamins, including thiamine, niacin and riboflavin.

1 1/2 cups orzo
1/4 cup apple juice
3 tablespoons white wine vinegar
2 tablespoons plus 2 teaspoons
   vegetable oil
2 teaspoons Dijon-style mustard
1/2 teaspoon ground ginger

1/2 teaspoon pepper
Pinch of salt
1/2 pound cherry tomatoes, halved
1 cup cooked black beans
  (1/2 cup dried)
1 cup cooked green peas
1 large yellow bell pepper, diced

Bring a medium-size saucepan of water to a boil. Add the orzo and cook for 8 to 10 minutes, or according to the package directions until al dente. Transfer the orzo to a colander, cool under cold running water and set aside to drain.

  In a medium-size bowl combine the apple juice, vinegar, oil, mustard, ginger, pepper and salt, and stir to combine. Add the tomatoes, beans, peas, bell pepper and orzo, and stir to combine. Serve the salad at room temperature or chilled.

Makes 6 servings

CALORIES per serving	327
66% Carbohydrate	55 g
14% Protein	11 g
20% Fat	7 g
CALCIUM	45 mg
IRON	3 mg
SODIUM	81 mg

STUFFED TROUT

Trout is a good source of omega-3 fatty acids, now recognized as useful in helping to reduce blood cholesterol levels.

1/2 cup low-sodium chicken stock
2 tablespoons butter
2 cups diced red bell peppers
1 1/2 cups sliced mushrooms
1 cup corn kernels
1 cup sliced yellow squash

1 cup chopped scallions
2 garlic cloves, chopped
5 cups whole-wheat bread cubes
One 1 1/2-pound brook
   trout, cleaned
1 lemon

Preheat the oven to 400° F. For the stuffing, bring the stock to a boil in a large skillet over medium-high heat. Add the butter, bell peppers, mushrooms, corn, squash, scallions and garlic, and cook, stirring constantly, until the mixture returns to a boil. Remove the skillet from the heat and stir in the bread until thoroughly combined; set aside.

   Rinse the trout and pat it dry with paper towels. Transfer three fourths of the stuffing to a large, shallow baking pan and pat it into an even layer. Place the trout on top and fill the cavity of the fish with the remaining stuffing. Cover the pan with foil and bake for 20 to 25 minutes, or until the fish flakes when tested with a fork. Halve the lemon and squeeze the juice of one half over the trout; slice the other half and use it to garnish the fish.   ·   Makes 4 servings

CALORIES per serving	317
44% Carbohydrate	37 g
29% Protein	24 g
27% Fat	10 g
CALCIUM	85 mg
IRON	4 mg
SODIUM	357 mg

Stuffed Trout

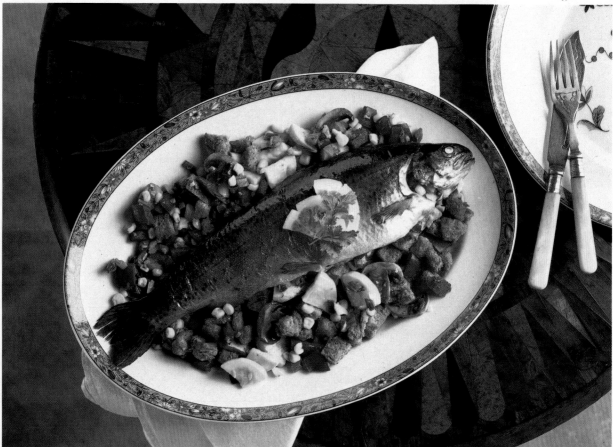

TURKEY SANDWICH WITH CRANBERRY CHUTNEY ▼

Lean turkey breast is one of the lowest-calorie choices for a meat sandwich. The homemade chutney has much less sugar than canned cranberry sauce, which may have as many as 12 teaspoons of sugar per serving.

CALORIES per serving	244
63% Carbohydrate	41 g
23% Protein	15 g
14% Fat	4 g
CALCIUM	95 mg
IRON	3 mg
SODIUM	293 mg

1 small apple, washed and cored
1 small seedless orange, washed
1/2 cup cranberries
2 teaspoons sugar
1 cup sliced mushrooms
8 slices whole-wheat bread
1 tablespoon whipped margarine

1/4 pound thinly sliced
  cooked turkey breast
1 cup grated carrots
2 tomatoes, sliced
2 cups Romaine lettuce, torn into
  bite-size pieces

For the chutney, cut the apple and orange into large chunks and place them in a food processor or blender. Add the cranberries and sugar, and process, pulsing the machine on and off, for about 20 seconds, or until the fruit is coarsely chopped and blended; set aside. In a small nonstick skillet cook the mushrooms with 1 tablespoon of water over medium heat, stirring often, for 3 to 5 minutes, or until softened.

Spread one side of each slice of bread with margarine. Divide the turkey among 4 slices of bread and top it with mushrooms, carrots, tomatoes and lettuce. Spread the remaining slices of bread with chutney and place them on top of the sandwiches. (If making the sandwiches ahead of time, do not add the chutney until just before serving, or it will soak through the bread.) Cut the sandwiches in half and serve immediately.   Makes 4 servings

PEACH AND OATMEAL CRISP

Heavy pastry and whipped cream can turn fruit into a high-fat dessert. Try this crisp oatmeal crust and yogurt topping instead. An added dividend: The fiber found in oats has been shown to lower blood cholesterol.

2 cups fresh or frozen
  unsweetened peach slices
1/4 cup dried currants
1 tablespoon honey
1/4 teaspoon ground cinnamon
1/4 teaspoon vanilla extract
1 cup rolled oats

3 tablespoons unbleached
  all-purpose flour
1 1/2 teaspoons light brown sugar
4 teaspoons butter or margarine
1 cup plain lowfat yogurt
1 teaspoon orange juice

> *An occasional indulgence in gourmet foods can help you stick to your low-calorie diet by keeping you from feeling deprived. Oysters are an example of such a food with outstanding nutritional benefits: They provide good amounts of iron, copper and zinc, contain cholesterol-lowering fish oil and have only about 10 calories each.*

Preheat the oven to 325° F. Reserving 8 thin peach slices for the garnish, combine the remaining peaches, the currants, honey, cinnamon and vanilla in a medium-size bowl, then spread the mixture evenly in an 8-inch square pan. For the topping, in a small bowl stir together the oats, flour and sugar, then work in the butter with your fingers until the mixture is crumbly. Sprinkle the topping over the peaches and bake for 45 minutes, or until the topping is browned. Let the crisp cool for 5 minutes. Meanwhile, for the topping stir together the yogurt and orange juice in a small bowl. Divide the peach crisp among 4 plates and top each serving with 1/4 cup of the yogurt mixture and 2 of the reserved peach slices.   Makes 4 servings

CALORIES per serving	273
70% Carbohydrate	49 g
11% Protein	8 g
19% Fat	6 g
CALCIUM	135 mg
IRON	2 mg
SODIUM	86 mg

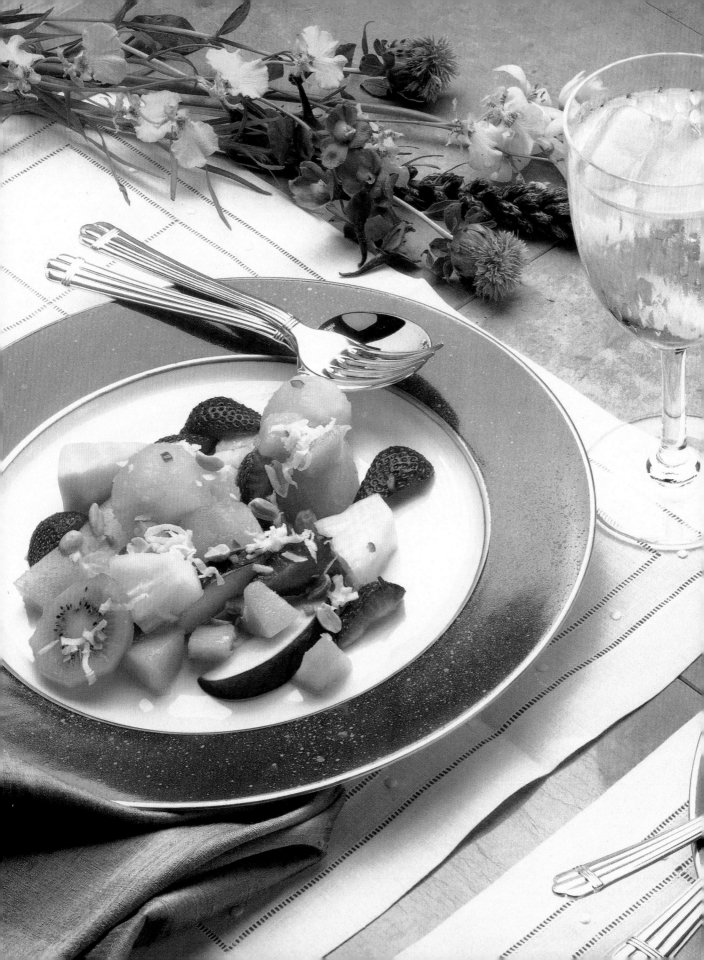

INDONESIAN-STYLE FRUIT SALAD

Even with coconut and peanuts (traditional Indonesian ingredients), this salad still derives less than 16 percent of its calories from fat. It is also an exceptional source of potassium and vitamins A and C.

CALORIES per serving	344
79% Carbohydrate	75 g
5% Protein	5 g
16% Fat	7 g
CALCIUM	81 mg
IRON	2 mg
SODIUM	28 mg

1 small jalapeño pepper, finely chopped

1/4 cup freshly squeezed lime juice

3 tablespoons honey

2 medium-size Delicious apples (3/4 pound total weight)

1 small honeydew melon

2 pints fresh strawberries

4 kiwi fruits

2 medium-size mangoes

4 cups fresh pineapple chunks, or juice-packed pineapple chunks, drained

1/2 cup shredded fresh or packaged unsweetened coconut

1/4 cup chopped roasted peanuts

For the dressing, in a small bowl combine the jalapeño with 3 tablespoons of lime juice and the honey; set aside. Core but do not peel the apples and cut them into 1/2-inch cubes. Place them in a small bowl and toss with the remaining lime juice. Cut the honeydew melon into balls or 1-inch cubes; you should have about 4 cups. Place the melon in a large bowl. Wash, hull and quarter the strawberries and add them to the bowl. Peel the kiwi fruits and mangoes, cut them into bite-size pieces and add them to the bowl. Add the apples, pineapple and dressing and toss well. Divide the salad among 6 plates, sprinkle with coconut and peanuts and serve.   Makes 6 servings

CALORIES per serving	97
51% Carbohydrate	13 g
18% Protein	5 g
31% Fat	4 g
CALCIUM	141 mg
IRON	3 mg
SODIUM	112 mg

P*arsley, often used as a garnish, is an underrated source of nutrients. A half-cup — just 32 calories' worth — fulfills your daily requirement for vitamins A and C, and supplies good amounts of iron, calcium and potassium. To increase your consumption of fresh parsley, think of it as a vegetable: Add the coarsely chopped leaves to green salads, tuna or chicken salad, or stir them into soups and sauces.*

CALORIES per serving	373
64% Carbohydrate	59 g
16% Protein	14 g
20% Fat	8 g
CALCIUM	53 mg
IRON	4 mg
SODIUM	274 mg

CREAMED SPINACH WITH ONIONS

Serve this vegetable mixture as a side dish, or make it a light meal by doubling the portion and having some whole-grain bread with it.

1 pound spinach, washed
  and trimmed
1 tablespoon butter
2 cups finely chopped onions

2 tablespoons unbleached
  all-purpose flour
1/2 cup skim milk
1/2 teaspoon ground nutmeg
1/4 teaspoon pepper

Bring 1 cup of water to a boil in a medium-size saucepan over medium-high heat. Add the spinach, and cook, stirring constantly, for 1 to 2 minutes, or until the spinach is wilted. Transfer the spinach to a colander and cool under cold running water. Drain and squeeze the excess water from the spinach. Finely chop the spinach; set aside. Rinse and dry the saucepan.

Melt the butter in the saucepan over medium heat, add the onions, and cook, stirring, for 1 minute. Add the flour and cook, stirring constantly, for another 2 minutes. Gradually add the milk and continue to cook and stir for 2 to 3 minutes more, or until the sauce is thick and smooth. Add the spinach, nutmeg and pepper, and cook, stirring, for another 2 to 3 minutes, or until the spinach is heated through. *Makes 4 servings*

PILAF WITH MARINATED FLANK STEAK

Flank steak is one of the leanest cuts of beef, with less fat than porterhouse or T-bone steak. Although marinating helps tenderize it, flank steak cannot be cooked beyond the medium-rare stage without toughening.

2 teaspoons vegetable oil
1 teaspoon lemon juice
1 teaspoon reduced-sodium
  soy sauce
1 teaspoon minced fresh ginger
1 teaspoon minced garlic
5 ounces lean flank steak
1 cup low-sodium chicken stock

1 1/3 cups white rice
2 cups broccoli florets
8 canned water chestnuts,
  drained and sliced
1/3 cup sliced scallions
2 teaspoons margarine
1/4 teaspoon salt
Pepper

In a small nonreactive bowl, stir together the oil, lemon juice, soy sauce, ginger and garlic. Add the steak, cover the bowl and set aside in a cool place to marinate for 1 hour, or refrigerate for at least 2 hours.

About 30 minutes before serving, bring the stock and 1 2/3 cups of water to a boil in a medium-size saucepan over medium-high heat. Stir in the rice, cover the pan, reduce the heat to low and simmer for 20 minutes, or until the rice is tender and the water is completely absorbed. Meanwhile, steam the broccoli in a vegetable steamer over boiling water for 5 minutes, or until tender; set aside. When the rice is done, stir in the broccoli, water chestnuts, scallions, margarine, salt, and pepper to taste; cover the pan and keep warm.

Preheat the broiler. Broil the steak for 4 minutes on each side, brushing it with the marinade as it cooks. Cut the steak against the grain into 1/4-inch-thick slices and serve it with the pilaf. *Makes 4 servings*

SOPA SECA

This Mexican sopa seca (dry soup) is a combination of pasta, shrimp and vegetables. A serving provides 4 grams of iron and plenty of vitamin C to aid in the absorption of iron.

1 cup low-sodium chicken stock

2 garlic cloves, chopped

1/2 teaspoon dried oregano

1/4 teaspoon red pepper flakes

1/8 teaspoon black pepper

7 ounces medium-size
  unshelled shrimp

2 cups diced green bell peppers

2 cups chopped onions

One 14-ounce can plum tomatoes

1/2 pound vermicelli, broken into
  2-inch pieces (2 cups)

3 tablespoons chopped
  fresh coriander

CALORIES per serving	327
69% Carbohydrate	56 g
25% Protein	20 g
6% Fat	2 g
CALCIUM	98 mg
IRON	4 mg
SODIUM	267 mg

In a large skillet bring 2 cups of water, the stock, garlic, oregano, red pepper and black pepper to a boil over medium heat. Add the shrimp and bell peppers and cook for 3 minutes, or until the shrimp turn bright pink. Using a slotted spoon, remove the shrimp and bell peppers; set aside. Add the onions and the tomatoes with their liquid to the soup and return to a boil over medium-high heat. Add the vermicelli, and cook, stirring frequently, for 8 to 10 minutes, or until it is tender. Return the shrimp and bell peppers to the pan, then stir in the coriander and serve. Makes 4 servings

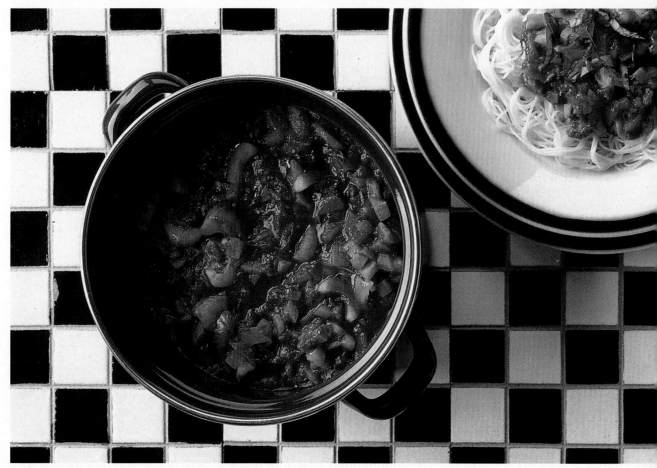

Crab Capellini

CRAB CAPELLINI

Pasta is an excellent calorie-watcher's meal if you keep the sauce low in fat.

CALORIES per serving	372
65% Carbohydrate	61 g
21% Protein	20 g
14% Fat	6 g
CALCIUM	137 mg
IRON	4 mg
SODIUM	481 mg

1 tablespoon olive oil
1 1/2 cups chopped onions
2 garlic cloves, chopped
Two 14-ounce cans plum tomatoes
1 cup chopped celery
3/4 cup chopped carrots

2 tablespoons chopped fresh basil
1 bay leaf
1/2 pound dried capellini
  or spaghetti
1/2 pound lump crabmeat
Black pepper

Heat the oil in a medium-size saucepan over medium heat. Add the onions and garlic, and sauté for 5 minutes, or until golden. Add the tomatoes and their liquid, the celery, carrots, 1 teaspoon of basil and the bay leaf, and bring to a boil. Reduce the heat to low and simmer the mixture, partially covered, for 30 minutes, or until the flavors are blended and the sauce is thickened.

Fifteen minutes before serving, bring a large pot of water to a boil. Cook the capellini for 8 to 10 minutes, or according to the package directions until al dente. Drain the pasta well and divide it among 4 plates. Place one fourth of the crabmeat on each portion and top it with the sauce. Sprinkle the sauce with pepper to taste and garnish with the reserved basil.   Makes 4 servings

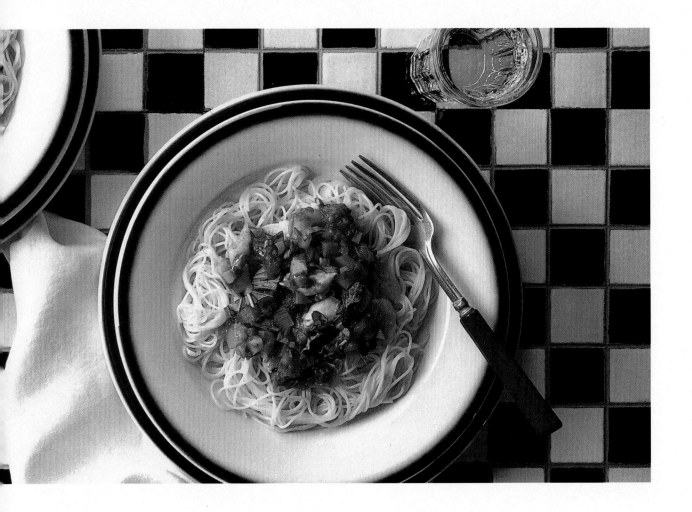

GINGER CHICKEN SOUP ▼

Serve this Oriental-style soup as a first course, or by itself as a light meal. Prepared without the use of any cooking oil or fat, the soup derives only 10 percent of its calories from fat.

CALORIES per serving	256
61% Carbohydrate	37 g
29% Protein	17 g
10% Fat	3 g
CALCIUM	123 mg
IRON	4 mg
SODIUM	102 mg

5 cups low-sodium chicken stock
3 cups shredded Chinese cabbage
1 large red bell pepper, cut into
   thin strips (1 1/2 cups)
1/4 pound fresh shiitake
   mushrooms, trimmed and sliced
1 cup thinly sliced scallions
2 tablespoons grated fresh ginger

1/4 pound chicken breast,
   cut into thin strips
6 ounces soba (Japanese
   buckwheat noodles), cooked
   and drained
3 cups chopped watercress leaves
1 tablespoon Japanese
   rice-wine vinegar

Bring the stock to a simmer in a large saucepan over medium-high heat. Add the cabbage, bell pepper, mushrooms, scallions and ginger, and simmer for another 5 minutes. Add the chicken and simmer the soup for 5 minutes more. Stir in the noodles, watercress and vinegar, and cook for another 2 minutes. Ladle the soup into 4 bowls and serve.   Makes 4 servings

CHICKEN POT PIE

Decorative pastry cutouts take the place of a full crust atop this vegetable-filled chicken stew, keeping fat and calories low.

CALORIES per serving	315
58% Carbohydrate	47 g
20% Protein	16 g
22% Fat	8 g
CALCIUM	62 mg
IRON	3 mg
SODIUM	142 mg

1/2 cup unbleached all-purpose flour, approximately

Pinch of salt

2 tablespoons chopped fresh dill

2 tablespoons butter, well chilled

1 tablespoon ice water

1 cup low-sodium chicken stock

3 cups unpeeled, diced new potatoes

1 cup chopped onions

3 cups broccoli florets

1 cup corn kernels

1 tablespoon cornstarch

1/4 pound skinless cooked chicken breast, cut into large chunks

In a small bowl stir together the flour, salt and 1 tablespoon of dill. Cut in the butter with a pastry blender or two knives until the mixture resembles coarse cornmeal. Add the ice water and stir until the dough forms a ball. Cover the bowl with a kitchen towel and set aside.

Bring the stock to a boil in a medium-size saucepan over medium heat. Add the potatoes and onions and return the mixture to a boil. Reduce the heat to medium-low, cover the pan and simmer the vegetables for 10 to 15 minutes, or until the potatoes are tender when pierced with a knife.

Preheat the oven to 400° F. Uncover the pan, add the broccoli and corn and return the mixture to a boil. In a small bowl stir together the cornstarch and 1/4 cup of cold water until smooth. Add the chicken to the saucepan, then stir in the cornstarch mixture and simmer for 1 to 2 minutes, or until the sauce thickens. Turn the chicken, vegetables and sauce into a shallow 10-inch baking dish and set aside.

Lightly flour a work surface and rolling pin. With your hands, flatten the dough into a disk, then roll it out 1/4 inch thick. Using a sharp knife, cut out a decorative chicken shape. (You may find it easier to make a cardboard pattern first.) Or cut small shapes from the dough with cookie cutters. Place the cut-out dough on top of the chicken mixture and bake for 15 to 20 minutes, or until the pastry is golden.   Makes 4 servings

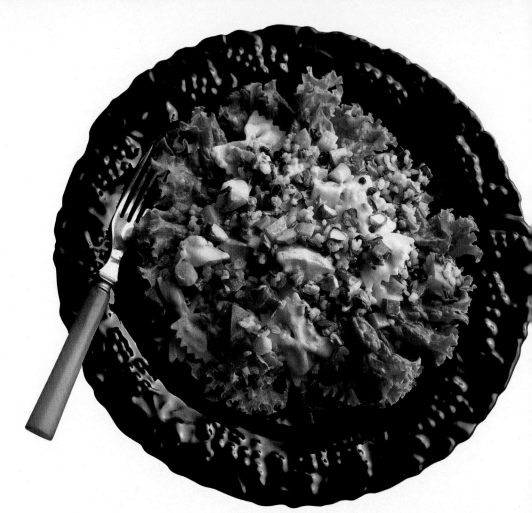

Two-Rice and Pasta Salad

TWO-RICE AND PASTA SALAD

Grains, pasta, fruit and nuts make this a satisfying main-dish salad.

CALORIES per serving	366
77% Carbohydrate	73 g
11% Protein	10 g
12% Fat	5 g
CALCIUM	115 mg
IRON	4 mg
SODIUM	474 mg

2 tablespoons dried currants
3/4 teaspoon salt
1/2 cup wild rice
1/2 cup brown rice
1 3/4 ounces small bow-tie pasta
  (about 1/2 cup)
3/4 pound Bosc pears
2 tablespoons lemon juice
1/4 cup lowfat sour cream

1/4 cup lowfat milk (2%)
2 tablespoons chutney
2 teaspoons curry powder
1 cup diced red bell peppers
1 cup diced carrots
1/2 cup chopped scallions
8 large lettuce leaves
3/4 ounce shelled, toasted
  pistachios (about 1/4 cup)

Place the currants in a small bowl with hot water to cover; set aside. Bring 2 quarts of water to a boil in a large saucepan over medium-high heat. Add 1/4 teaspoon of salt, the wild rice and brown rice, and cook, stirring occasionally, for 40 minutes. Add the pasta and cook for 8 minutes. Drain the rice and pasta in a large strainer, cool under cold water and set aside to drain.

  Core the pears, cut them into 3/4-inch cubes and place them in a bowl. Add the lemon juice and toss well. For the dressing, in a small bowl combine the sour cream, milk, chutney, curry powder, the remaining salt and 1 tablespoon of the lemon juice from the bowl of pears. In a large bowl combine the rice and pasta with the bell peppers, carrots, scallions, pears and currants. Add the dressing and toss well, then cover the bowl and refrigerate until well chilled.

To serve, line 4 plates with lettuce leaves and mound the salad on top. Sprinkle the salad with pistachios and serve.   Makes 4 servings

SCALLOP BISQUE

The soup is extremely rich in nutrients, with more potassium than two bananas, more vitamin C than two oranges, more calcium than a cup of whole milk and more iron than a cup of prune juice.

1 tablespoon vegetable oil	1 cup sliced mushrooms
3 tablespoons unbleached all-purpose flour	2 ounces bay scallops
	2 tablespoons lowfat sour cream
1/4 cup minced shallots	1 1/2 teaspoons grated lemon peel
2 cups skim milk	1/4 teaspoon salt
1/2 cup low-sodium chicken stock	Black pepper
1 cup grated carrots	2 tablespoons chopped fresh parsley
1 cup each diced red and yellow bell pepper	

CALORIES per serving	323
47% Carbohydrate	39 g
22% Protein	18 g
31% Fat	11 g
CALCIUM	350 mg
IRON	4 mg
SODIUM	498 mg

Heat the oil in a large saucepan over medium heat. Add the flour and shallots, and cook, stirring, for 2 minutes. Do not let the flour brown. Whisk in the milk, stock and 1/2 cup of water and continue whisking until smooth. Add the carrots, bell peppers and mushrooms and bring the mixture to a boil, then reduce the heat to low and simmer the soup for 15 minutes, or until the vegetables are tender. Transfer the soup to a food processor or blender and process until puréed. Return the soup to the saucepan, add the scallops and cook over medium-low heat for 5 minutes, or until the scallops are opaque. Stir in the sour cream, lemon peel, salt, and pepper to taste, and ladle the soup into 2 bowls. Sprinkle with parsley and serve.   Makes 2 servings

GINGERED SQUASH AND CABBAGE

The appetizing contrast of crisp Napa (a type of Chinese cabbage) and creamy squash in this side dish can enliven a simple lowfat meal.

1 butternut squash	3 cups Napa cabbage, cut into 1/4-inch-wide strips
3 garlic cloves	
1 cup low-sodium chicken stock	4 ounces fresh shiitake mushrooms, trimmed and sliced
3 thick slices fresh ginger	

CALORIES per serving	67
80% Carbohydrate	15 g
16% Protein	3 g
4% Fat	3 g
CALCIUM	97 mg
IRON	1 mg
SODIUM	23 mg

Peel and seed the squash and cut it into 1/4-inch-thick slices. Crush and peel the garlic. Bring the stock to a boil in a medium-size saucepan over medium heat. Add the garlic and ginger, reduce the heat to low, cover and simmer for 10 minutes. Remove and discard the garlic and ginger. Add the cabbage, squash and mushrooms, cover the pan and simmer, stirring occasionally, for another 10 minutes, or until the vegetables are tender.   Makes 4 servings

141

PROP CREDITS

Cover: sweat pants–The Gap, San Francisco, Calif.; page 6: leotard–Danskin, Inc., New York City; page 42: orange juicer, toaster, mug–The Pottery Barn, New York City; page 50: plates–The Pottery Barn, New York City; page 53: rug–Cobweb Antique Imports, New York City; pages 54-55: plates, bowl–The Hall China Co., East Liverpool, Ohio; page 58: plate–Platypus, New York City; bowl–Mood Indigo, New York City, linens–Ad Hoc Softwares, New York City; plate, cup and saucer, salt and pepper courtesy of Nola Lopez, New York City, napkin–Ad Hoc Softwares, New York City; page 65–checkered bowl, dark blue plate–The Pottery Barn, New York City, purple plate–Mood Indigo, New York City; pages 66-67: Fiesta plates, cup and saucer, pitcher, salt and pepper–The Homer Laughlin China Co., courtesy of D. King Irwin, Inc., New York City, flatware, glasses–Mood Indigo, New York City, tablecloth courtesy of Charles Rizzuto, New York City; page 68: plate, spoon–Frank MacIntosh at Henri Bendel, New York City, napkin–Ad Hoc Softwares, New York City, tile–Ceramique Francois, New York City; page 73: plates–Ad Hoc Softwares, New York City; page 92-93: plates, flatware–Saski, New York City, glasses–Frank MacIntosh at Henri Bendel, New York City, flamingo salt and pepper courtesy of Dean Morris, New York City; page 95: bowl–Lanie Cecula, courtesy of Contemporary Porcelain, New York City; page 96: plates, glasses–Amigo Country, New York City, linens–Ad Hoc Softwares, New York City, cactus salt and pepper courtesy of Valorie Fisher, New York City; page 98-99: white plate–Lone Oak& Co., courtesy of Platypus, New York City; page 102: platter–Mood Indigo, New York City; page 105: plates, cup and saucer–Mood Indigo, New York City, spoon, linens courtesy of Nola Lopez, New York City; page 106: wood bowls–Zona, New York City; page 108: tote bag–The Pottery Barn, New York City; page 116: plate–Marek and Lanie Cecula, courtesy of Contemporary Porcelain, New York City, glass–Platypus, New York City; pages 118-119: terra-cotta plates, glass–Gear, New York City, gray plate, concrete bowl–Sointu, New York City, flatware, straw mat–The Pottery Barn, New York City, salt shaker courtesy of Nola Lopez, New York City; page 121: plates, bowl–Daniel Levy Ceramics, New York City, linens–Ad Hoc Softwares, New York City, salt and pepper–Swid Powell, New York City, tile–Ceramique Francois, New York City; page 122: plate, glass–Gear, New York City, flatware–Puiforcat, courtesy of Baccarat, Inc., New York City, linens–Ad Hoc Softwares, New York City; page 126: bowl, plate, spoon–Frank MacIntosh at Henri Bendel, New York City; page 129: bowl–Lanie Cecula, courtesy of Contemporary Porcelain, New York City, plate, glass–Frank MacIntosh at Henri Bendel, New York City, flatware–Puiforcat, courtesy of Baccarat, Inc., New York City; page 130: plates–Raynaud Ceralene, courtesy of Bac-carat, Inc., New York City, table courtesy of Martha and Robert Weisberg, New York City; pages 132-133: plates, glasses, flatware–Baccarat, Inc., New York City, linens–Ad Hoc Softwares, New York City, tile–Ceramique Francois, New York City; page 135: plate, glass, flatware–Baccarat, Inc., linens–Ad Hoc Softwares, New York City, tile–Ceramique Francois, New York City; pages 136-137: plates–Buffalo China, Inc., Buffalo, N.Y., tile–Country Floors, Inc., New York City; pages 138-139: plate, tablecloth courtesy of Nola Lopez, New York City; page 140: plate–Gear, New York City.

ACKNOWLEDGMENTS

All cosmetics and grooming products supplied by Clinique Labs, Inc., New York City

Nutrition analysis provided by Hill Nutrition Associates, Fayette-ville, N.Y.

Off-camera warm-up equipment: rowing machine supplied by Precor USA, Redmond, Wash.; Tunturi stationary bicycle supplied by Amerec Corp., Bellevue, Wash.

Washing machine and dryer supplied by White-Westinghouse, Columbus, Ohio

Index prepared by Ian Tucker

Production by Giga Communications

PHOTOGRAPHY CREDIT

All photographs by Steven Mays, Rebus, Inc.

ILLUSTRATION CREDITS

Page 8, illustration: Tammi Colichio; page 11, illustration: Tammi Colichio; page 12, illustration: David Flaherty; page 15, illustration: David Flaherty; page 16, illustration: Tammi Colichio; page 18, illustration: David Flaherty; page 21, illustration: Tammi Colichio; page 25, chart: Brian Sisco; page 26, illustration: Tammi Colichio; page 31, illustration: Brian Sisco; pages 34-35, chart: Brian Sisco; pages 36-37, chart: Brian Sisco; page 39, chart: Brian Sisco; page 41, chart: Brian Sisco; page 47, chart: Brian Sisco; pages 48-49, illustration: David Flaherty; page 79, chart: Brian Sisco; page 81, illustration: Tammi Colichio; page 113, chart: Brian Sisco; page 114, illustration: David Flaherty; page 115, illustration: David Flaherty.

Time-Life Books Inc. offers a wide range of fine recordings, including a Rock 'n' Roll Era series. For subscription information, call 1-800-621-7026, or write TIME-LIFE MUSIC, P. O. Box C-32068; Richmond, Virginia 23261-2068.

INDEX